Cultivating Health

Critical Issues in Health and Medicine

Edited by Rima D. Apple, University of Wisconsin–Madison,
and Janet Golden, Rutgers University, Camden

Growing criticism of the U.S. healthcare system is coming from consumers, politicians, the media, activists, and healthcare professionals. Critical Issues in Health and Medicine is a collection of books that explores these contemporary dilemmas from a variety of perspectives, among them political, legal, historical, sociological, and comparative, and with attention to crucial dimensions such as race, gender, ethnicity, sexuality, and culture.

For a list of titles in the series, see the last page of the book.

Cultivating Health

Los Angeles Women and Public Health Reform

Jennifer Lisa Koslow

Rutgers University Press
New Brunswick, New Jersey, and London

Library of Congress Cataloging-in-Publication Data

Koslow, Jennifer Lisa, 1970–
   Cultivating health : Los Angeles women and public health reform / Jennifer Lisa Koslow.
      p. ; cm.—(Critical issues in health and medicine)
   Includes bibliographical references and index.
   ISBN 978-0-8135-4528-8 (hardcover : alk. paper)
   1. Health care reform—California—Los Angeles—History—20th century. 2. Health care reform—California—Los Angeles—History—20th century. 3. Women health reformers—California—Los Angeles—History—19th century. I. Title. II. Series.
   [DNLM: 1. Health Care Reform—history—Los Angeles. 2. Public Health—history—Los Angeles. 3. History, 20th Century—Los Angeles. 4. Maternal Health Services—history—Los Angeles. 5. Public Health Nursing—history—Los Angeles. 6. Sanitation—history—Los Angeles. 7. Women—history—Los Angeles. WA 11 AC2 K86c 2009]
   RA395.A4C2765 2009
   362.1'04250979494—dc22
                                                                                                        2008048061

A British Cataloging-in-Publication record for this book is available from the British Library.

Copyright © 2009 by Jennifer Lisa Koslow

All rights reserved

No part of this book may be reproduced or utilized in any form or by any means, electronic or mechanical, or by any information storage and retrieval system, without written permission from the publisher. Please contact Rutgers University Press, 100 Joyce Kilmer Avenue, Piscataway, NJ 08854–8099. The only exception to this prohibition is "fair use" as defined by U.S. copyright law.

Visit our Web site: http://rutgerspress.rutgers.edu

Manufactured in the United States of America

For Patrick

Contents

	Preface and Acknowledgments	ix
	Introduction	1
Chapter 1	Paid for by the Public Purse: Public Health Nursing	10
Chapter 2	Public Authority for a Private Program: Housing Reform	44
Chapter 3	Bovines, Babies, and Bacteriology: The Problems of Crafting Milk Reform	77
Chapter 4	Delivering the City's Children: Midwives and Municipal Maternity Programs	104
Chapter 5	The Challenge of Constructing Venereal Disease Programs	132
	Conclusion	156
	List of Abbreviations	161
	Notes	163
	Index	195

Preface and Acknowledgments

On a cold and blustery Chicago day, the public health nurse trudged up three flights of stairs carrying her black bag. Behind her followed an assistant bearing a large analog baby scale. A premature birth of twins prompted the visit. She came to check on their progress and that of their mother. The twins were undressed, weighed, and their limbs and torsos were examined. A bell was rung next to one ear and then the other, and a red ball of yarn danced above their heads. They passed these simple tests. They could hear, see, and had gained weight since leaving the hospital. Next, the nurse asked the mother to fill out a form regarding her state of mind. She also appeared to pass the test. If the family were not moving out-of-state in a few weeks, the visiting nurse would have returned to check on everyone's health.

When I began this project I never imagined that I would have such an intimate encounter with the legacy of the reforms I studied. I also never imagined that I would give birth to twins. So when I had the opportunity to merge my personal and professional lives, I took it. I have to admit that the first phone call from the public health nurse was a bit off-putting. After having been through a nerve-wracking couple of weeks I was unprepared to have a member of the health department leave a message on my machine asking to speak with me. Why? Did my children have some disease that had only shown up in tests sent to the state? How did the city get my number? All this became clear in speaking with the nurse. The hospital alerted the city about the twins' premature birth and, in particular, about the early episodes of apnea in one of them. She asked for permission to pay us a visit. While I had the advantage of access to private medical care, I was more than a bit curious and welcomed her into our home.

In some ways the encounter differed quite greatly from my studies. Sitting around my dining room table were a mix of ethnicities that would never have been put together in this type of power arrangement by reformers in the early twentieth century. The nurse was Indian, her assistant was African American, and their patients were white. The nurse also made an appointment rather than just showing up at our doorstep. In some ways, however, I suspect she would have recognized some of the techniques used by her early-twentieth-century peers. Her low-tech devices for determining health differed dramatically from the high-tech world the twins and their parents had become quickly accustomed to in the Neonatal Intensive Care Unit. Yet, they were no less effective.

The nurse's calm demeanor led us to greatly appreciate her knowledge, skill, and attention.

Though we had no more encounters, I can only imagine that if we had stayed I would have looked forward to more visits. It was nice to have someone come to us rather than bundle the babies and venture out into the cold. It was also reassuring to know that someone was checking on our well-being. What if I did not have health insurance? What if I did not have a car to bring my babies to their pediatrician? In a time when the direction of health care seems to be moving ever more toward privatization, I find comfort in the city's continued commitment to provide for the health of its residents. What follows is the story of how the state came to realize its responsibility for protecting and promoting the public's health.

Without the generous support of others, I would not have been able to complete this work. I have been fortunate to receive financial support from the National Library of Medicine/National Institutes of Health (Grant #1-G13-LM008430-01), the Huntington Library, the American Historical Association, the Historical Society of Southern California, the UCLA History Department, the UCLA Center for the Study of Women, and Florida State University. While I have received the kind help of archivists too numerous to mention, I especially want to thank Katherine Donahue and Teresa Johnson of the UCLA Louise M. Darling Biomedical Library's History and Special Collections for the Sciences and the current and former Los Angeles City archivists Jay Jones and Hynda Rudd.

Portions of chapters 3 and 4 initially appeared, in slightly different form, in the following publications, and I am grateful to the publishers for permission to include them here: "Putting It to a Vote: The Provision of Pure Milk in Progressive Era Los Angeles," *The Journal of the Gilded Age and Progressive Era*, Volume 3, no. 2 (2004): 111–144; "Delivering the City's Children: Municipal Programs and Midwifery in Los Angeles," *Canadian Bulletin of Medical History*, Volume 19, 2 (2002): 399–443. I also wish to acknowledge the editors of *The Development of Los Angeles City Government: An Institutional History, 1850–2000* (Los Angeles City Historical Society, 2007) for allowing reproduction of portions from my contribution to that work.

On the road to publication, I have accrued numerous debts. To Jan Reiff, I owe my deepest appreciation for her sound advice and invaluable comments these many years. My sincerest thanks to Toby Higbie for his intellectual insights and friendship. I also owe a debt of gratitude to Emily Abel, Sara Austin, Rachel Bohlmann, Lynne Curry, Carolyn Eastman, Leon Fink, Maureen Flanagan, Robert G. Frank, James Grossman, Sally Hadden, Evelynn Hammonds, Robert

Johnston, Sarah Buck-Kachaluba, Richard R. John, Stephanie Leitch, Susan Levine, Doug Knox, Valerie Matsumoto, Darrin McMahon, Claudia Mineo, Sarah Pearsall, Heike Schmidt, Aaron Shapiro, Jeffrey Sklansky, Susan L. Smith, Charles Upchurch, Frank Valadez, and Alfred E. Young for taking the time to read various portions and offer comments. My thanks to all my colleagues at Florida State University; I'm enormously appreciative of your confidence in me. I am especially grateful for the guidance of Neil Jumonville, Elna Green, Suzy Sinke, and Fritz Davis. I also want to express thanks to my graduate assistants Tiffany Baker and Kim Hernandez. My sincerest appreciation to Janet Golden, Rima D. Apple, Ruth Crocker, the anonymous reviewer, and Doreen Valentine for their guidance in seeing this manuscript through its final stages.

Over the years, my friends and family have acquiesced as intellectual sounding boards and cheerful companions. My thanks to David Behin, Anastasia Christman, Veronica Coleman, Carla Copeland, Jane Dabel, Riva Feschbach, Loretta Gaffney, Bruce Gerstman, Julia Mass, Lisa Materson, Carrie Messenger, Heather McKay, Shelley McKay, Gail Ostergren, Roberta Rosen, Josh Sides, Mat Verna, and John Xavier. I am grateful to my mother and stepfather, Susan Rosen and Harold Olejarz, for their encouragement and support. I owe a debt of thanks to Mary Byrne and the late Nicholas C. Byrne, whose love and care packages have been life sustaining. To my big brother and fellow professor, Julian Koslow: I admire your intellect and humor. I thank my father, Arnold Koslow (the first Prof. Koslow), for his wisdom, laughter, patience, and for instilling in me the value of empathy. To Lillian and Ramona, you are my sunshines. To Patrick: standing on the moon, what a lovely view of heaven, but I'd rather be with you.

Cultivating Health

Introduction

In the early 1900s, most women experienced the rigors of childbirth at home. Whom could they call when complications occurred? In the case of a thirty-five-year-old Russian immigrant woman who failed to regain her strength two weeks after giving birth, her family did not call a physician or a midwife. Instead, they asked a social service agency, the Los Angeles College Settlement Association, to send a nurse. Upon arrival, the nurse assessed the patient as having "made a very poor recovery, was anemic, no appetite, and running a little temperature."[1] Following the protocol set forth by her supervisor, a reformer by the name of Maude Foster Weston, the nurse advocated sending the patient to the hospital. The family, however, "positively refused to allow" this. Their response probably did not surprise the nurse because aversion to hospitalization was a fairly typical response among the working class during this period.[2] Despite her supervisor's policy directives, the nurse revised her plan and called for a physician, who left medicines to be administered daily. Yet, the patient would not take the medication unless the nurse was present, leaving the family "very much dissatisfied" when the patient did not improve. The family's actions frustrated the nurse. She resolved the issue by threatening never to return "unless they would do as they were told." Presumably because they still wanted help, the family complied. According to the nurse's account, although it took "two months of hard work," she finally began to see a recovery. The nurse ended her report by stating "we have gained the confidence of the family and they know what was done was for the welfare of the patient." The nurse restored this patient's health but her assistance felt obtrusive and engendered suspicion.

The creation of social services at the turn of the twentieth century brought life-saving help into people's homes. It was also mainly the result of private, nongovernmental initiative. In the nineteenth century, cities did not have public health care systems. Instead they relied on medical practitioners in private practice and civic-minded citizens to donate their expertise and money in times of crisis. Women directed disaster response efforts whether it was attending to the sanitary conditions of military camps and hospitals during the Civil War or organizing relief for the residents of Chicago after a fire destroyed much of that city in 1871. By the end of the century, public health projects became reactions not only to catastrophic disaster but also to broader developments in the urbanization of America. Unchecked urban growth resulted in contaminated food supplies, substandard housing, and lack of access to medical care in many cities. In the absence of regulatory protections, working-class families were particularly vulnerable to quality of life questions. These environmental and social crises sparked a surge of reform across the nation, with women leading the way. They formulated professional responses. Yet, instead of rejecting a role for government in advancing an individual's everyday existence, female reformers embraced it. They laid the groundwork for the government's active participation in promoting the health of its citizens, especially for those most at risk. This stood in contrast to government's previous public health stance that was more limited in its nature.

By the end of the nineteenth century, citizens expected municipalities to shoulder the responsibility of taking care of the public's health during epidemics. The construction of large-scale sanitation projects, aqueducts, and sewer lines demonstrated cities' willingness to increase their civic capacities.[3] The primary justification given for funding these expensive ventures was the need to combat dirt, which was believed to be the origin of disease. The advent of the germ theory in the 1880s, while not immediately transformative, challenged society to revisit the question of personal accountability.[4] Throughout the early twentieth century, public health officials shifted their gaze from populations to individual people's hygienic habits. In this moment of transition, women seized the opportunity to develop the municipality's role even further. They advocated expanding access by routinely bringing public medical care into working people's homes to improve their standard of living.

Reformers argued that citizen volunteerism should be aimed at securing state responsibility. In other words, although reformers initially offered solutions for a city's public health woes, they planned on eventually transferring control of their agendas to officials. In the absence of a strong federal or state public health presence in the nineteenth century, the municipality became the site of state making. It was where citizens created political structures to produce social order.[5] Although the reformers' goal was to involve the government, the idea of public health that they wished to see implemented was not one that originated from government itself. Instead, their strategy was derived from and shaped by the complex exchanges that took place within immigrant working-class homes such as that anxious Russian family's domicile. Through these ordinary encounters, reformers, health professionals, and patients negotiated the implementation of public health policies. Out of such conflicted scenes arose a shared sense of the necessity of health care.

Middle-class women fostered this approach. They, rather than city officials, expanded the character of public health. The politics of health were also often contested by businessmen, private physicians, and the general public.[6] As public health policy teetered between balancing the interests of the general welfare with those of private individuals, it required many compromises and brought into play a variety of conceptual and ideological problems. In negotiating these compromises, for example, reformers paradoxically found maternalism—an ideology associating women with the home and family—to be an especially powerful tool for enabling women to engage public policy debates over extending government's role and citizen action.[7] These women asserted that, as women, they knew best how to nurture the city's poor. They used this idea to justify their involvement in transforming partisan politics, agitate for suffrage, police adolescent sexuality, and even engage in urban planning.[8] But this was not the only factor shaping these women's arguments or their outlook. Their beliefs about disease, urban space, racial prejudices, and class biases also influenced the ways in which they formed public health programs and, in turn, how these programs shaped social conditions within the city.[9]

Coping with unrestricted capitalist growth at the end of the nineteenth century prompted endeavors for restructuring throughout the United States, but nowhere was the impulse for reform stronger than in southern California. For instance, although American author Edward Bellamy's socialist utopian melodrama *Looking Backward* inspired thousands throughout the United States to join Nationalist clubs to discuss the ideas it raised and ways to realize its vision, 40 percent of these clubs were founded in California and over half of those were located in the southern region of the state.[10] Sometimes dubbed the quintessential "Progressive" city, Los Angeles was a leader in political and social reforms. In 1903, it became the first city to adopt the use of the referendum, initiative, and recall. Shortly thereafter, it outlawed vice and approved the prohibition of alcohol. Los Angelenas were particularly influential in securing the passage of suffrage in California almost a decade before the ratification of the Nineteenth Amendment in 1920. Why reform struck such a chord in Los Angeles remains elusive, but it was within this vibrant reform community that women appointed themselves as investigators and instigators on matters related to public health.[11]

Settled first by the Tongva, colonized by the Spanish in 1781, ceded to the Mexicans in 1821, and conquered by the Americans in 1848, Los Angeles experienced public health problems throughout its history. Until the 1880s, however, they were problems of the small town that Los Angeles was back then, rather than the large city it would become. In 1850, for instance, the city council managed public health and civic beautification by instructing every householder to clean the area from the front of his home to the middle of the street every Saturday.[12] A tremendous growth in population in the 1880s changed the dynamics of public health in Los Angeles. In that single decade the city's population jumped from 11,183 to 50,395, as tens of thousands of people were attracted to the 29-square-mile city by inexpensive railroad tickets, the promise of making a quick fortune in real estate, an abundance of jobs, and a belief that California's climate was curative. The combination of this demographic change and a smallpox epidemic in 1887 prompted the city to establish a permanent board of health, a health office, and a health officer when it rewrote its charter in 1889. Despite a brief bust at the end of the 1880s, Los Angeles continued to grow in population and in geographic territory throughout the early twentieth century. By 1930, Los Angeles had become the fifth most populous city in the United States, its population reaching over a million.

While city boosters sold Los Angeles as the "Land of Sunshine," living and working conditions did not always live up to such sunny promises.[13] Local public health records indicate that recent immigrant workers, whose labor sustained the city's industries of tourism and agribusiness, encountered conditions of poverty in Los Angeles similar to those experienced by their counterparts living in eastern and midwestern cities. Epidemiological studies linked rates of poverty to rates of sickness. These public health statistics were used to justify state control over lives and bodies.[14] Working-class immigrants became the subjects of public health scrutiny in Los Angeles and elsewhere. Out of empathy and fear, reformers and health professionals monitored immigrants' health, and their findings were used to justify immigration restrictions in the 1920s.[15]

Place and race played determining factors in public health. Despite the contemporary association of Los Angeles with sprawl, the city was fairly compact and its immigrant communities tended to live in close proximity to the central downtown area.[16] Mexicans, Japanese, Chinese, and southern and eastern European immigrants lived as neighbors. In distributing health care in this multicultural setting, public health officials and reformers exercised social power. Their governmental and nongovernmental public health programs were used to fasten racial distinctions. As a result, social services did not meet issues of health alone, but shaped and managed the social fabric of the city.

In spite of health efforts to keep up with the stresses of urban growth, residents of Los Angeles continued to experience epidemics of disease, exposure to dangerous living and working conditions, and problems providing access to health care. The most visible and visceral issue was mortality. Between 1890 and 1930, the city's mortality rate vacillated between eleven to fifteen deaths per thousand. While Los Angeles was not the deadliest city in the United States, this was still a worrisome statistic that indicated a significant level of risk. Health officials expressed concern over the numbers of deaths caused by tuberculosis, heart disease, cancer, pneumonia, and nephritis. While not nearly as statistically fatal, typhoid fever, measles, scarlet fever, whooping cough, and diphtheria remained diseases of concern because of their relatively high rates of incidence. More troubling was the city's infant mortality rate, which became a standard measure by which public health reformers judged the status of their cities; in 1889, Los Angeles's rate was 168 deaths per 1,000 live births. The same year, the health department estimated that zymotic (contagious) diseases caused 24 percent of all deaths in the city. Recalculating the numbers to include diseases that we now know are bacterial or viral in origin, contagious diseases caused at least 44 percent of all deaths in Los Angeles. With all this death and disease the city still lacked a municipal safety net.

In response, volunteer organizations took the lead in crafting health services for the city's poorer residents. Religious groups answered initial calls for citizen assistance. In 1854, a few Jewish men formed the Jewish Benevolent Society, making it the first organized charity group in the city. The Sisters of Charity, a Roman Catholic benevolence organization, created an infirmary in 1859. In the ensuing years, the Episcopal Church founded a hospital for noninfectious patients, and a number of other ethnic minorities set up benevolent associations. While some of these institutions were open to all people, such as the Sisters of Charity's infirmary, others were not. Wealth, ethnicity, religion, and race all served as restrictive factors. Hence, as the city developed, so did its segregated services.

The most important secular organization to provide public health services for the city's residents during the early twentieth century, the Los Angeles College Settlement Association, derived its origins from a women's social club. In 1891, white middle-class women began to meet every Friday morning to converse about culture and current events. Founded by Caroline Severance, "the Mother of Women's Clubs," the Friday Morning Club (FMC) was the oldest women's club in Los Angeles. Although technically a private club, in the 1890s, members could bring in three guests per quarter and special allowances were made for nonresident and male visitors. Thus, at certain moments the FMC functioned as a public forum for discussing contemporary social, economic, and political issues.[17] In the 1890s, members and their guests could learn about the "Property Rights of Married Women in California," watch Mrs. J. H. Patzki (employer) and Miss Wade (employee) debate "Domestic Service: How to Remove Prejudice Against It," or listen to Sara P. Monks describe "Studies with a Microscope."[18] By placing a diversity of topics on the agenda, the FMC could pique the curiosity of any member and, at the same time, legitimize women's claims to concerns beyond homemaking and the arts.

In retrospect, the FMC's meeting on February 2, 1894, was particularly important for instigating women's involvement in public health reform in Los Angeles, although by all initial appearances it was to have been a routine assembly. In the aftermath of the economic depression of 1893, FMC members met to discuss "The Unemployed." Sarah Longstreth provided statistics and Jennie E. Collier argued for "the sifting of the tramps from the workers," offering the latter relief through employment in public service and advocating the removal of protectionist tariffs to stimulate job growth.[19] Attracted by the issues on the agenda, representatives of the major local newspapers attended the event. Though they led their coverage with news about the planned program, the bulk of their reports focused on the unscheduled speeches made by the two visitors who spoke after Collier: Jane Addams and James B. Reynolds.

By 1894, Jane Addams and James B. Reynolds were both nationally renowned social reformers.[20] Described by the press as a "magnetic and delightful speaker" with "luminous eyes and fine face," Addams discussed the means by which the members of Hull House carried out public health work and educational projects in Chicago. Reynolds, whose physical features the reporters did not describe, was the head of the New York University Settlement. He decided to broach a more sensitive issue: local conditions. Depending on the journalistic source, either the women of the FMC asked Reynolds to offer his opinion on environmental circumstances in Los Angeles, or he volunteered his impression unsolicited. In either case, Reynolds asserted that the moral and physical state of Los Angeles was more deplorable than anything he had seen in the cities of Europe, Asia, and Africa. According to the *Los Angeles Herald* and the *Los Angeles Express*, Reynolds "urged" club members to "study" their city and to "plan for better conditions." The editors of the

Express responded by accusing Reynolds, "in the parlance of the street," of "talking through his hat."[21]

Within weeks of Addams's and Reynolds's visit, a small social group of women who had graduated from Wellesley, Vassar, Oberlin, and Northwestern, and had organized themselves into the Collegiate Alumni Association of Los Angeles, established the Los Angeles College Settlement Association (LACSA).[22] Although the archival record does not reveal whether these women were members of the FMC or had been at the meeting on February 2, 1894, they lived in the same social milieu.[23] A clipping from the *Los Angeles Times* indicates that FMC members Kate Tupper Galpin and Dorothea Lummis spoke about their visit to Hull House the previous summer with the alumnae just days before the February gathering.[24] Given the timing of proceedings, the public nature of the FMC's gathering, and these women's general interests, it is reasonable to infer that the alumnae found inspiration to create LACSA from the combination of these events.

By establishing a settlement house, these women joined a transatlantic movement for social reform.[25] The settlement functioned as a vehicle with which to inform the public structures responsible for shaping social conditions within the city.[26] LACSA was not the only organization of this type in Los Angeles, but it exerted the most direct influence on the health department.[27] It used its avowedly secular character to justify its clout over civic affairs. It was also the first female-dominated institution to pursue the strategy of creating public health programs for the city to incorporate. Each focus of reform (public health nursing, housing, and childbirth) became a specific bureau or division within the city's health department. LACSA laid the basis for clubwomen's pursuit of municipal milk reform and for social hygienists' civic programs for venereal disease treatment. Hence, while the settlement created only a few particular programs, these reveal the interconnections between women's diverse concerns and their translation into public policy. In this manner, health officers remained responsible for carrying out regulatory measures to prevent the spread of disease, but it was women who became the chief architects of civic programs for the promotion of health.

Female reformers in Los Angeles, like many other middle-class women across the nation, attempted to mitigate the dangers of turn-of-the-twentieth-century city life. As these women developed new understandings about the perils of urban living, they called attention to the diseases of domesticity. According to their worldview, bad housekeeping could be life threatening, and they deemed immigrant women as the most likely culprits. But, in engaging in public health reform in Los Angeles, women went beyond maternalism in search of other strategies. Science, especially microbiologic discoveries, offered an enticing alternative source of authority.[28] Their perception of Los Angeles as a "health Mecca" and the West as demographically unique prompted them to use microbiologic discoveries for activist purposes. Hence, they employed sympathy and science to agitate for reform.[29]

Yet, as they would later admit, even local settlement workers were sometimes blind to potential public health threats because the city did not conform to their expectations of urban space. Consequently, the encounter with Addams and Reynolds was not the last time they drew their muse from eastern and midwestern activists. A lecture by Jacob Riis, a photojournalist and best-selling author about New York City's slums, caused reformers to recognize that house courts in Los Angeles, while single storied and spread out, replicated tenement conditions of New York's Lower East Side. In much the same way, local women pondered whether the relatively close proximity of dairy farms guaranteed the purity of their milk supply only after being questioned by Florence Kelley, head of the National Consumer's League that worked to protect the dignity of labor and ensure the safety and quality of manufactures. Once their problems were pointed out by these visitors, however, they quickly modified eastern strategies to solve what they believed were western problems.

Although medical practitioners, public health professionals, and the public discover, describe, and redefine ailments depending upon the discourse of their day, parasites exist and exert biological impacts upon their hosts.[30] Consequently, although these women's perceptions of jeopardy were socially constructed, their fears cannot be dismissed as complete fabrication. Their reform efforts were a meaningful and effective practical endeavor in the face of genuine threat. Responding to disease presented real dilemmas to which the government initially held no answers.

Reformers in the East and Midwest often created structures parallel to city bureaucracies or, in time, leap-frogged over the local administration to turn to the state and federal government to protect the public's health. In contrast, women in Los Angeles persisted in focusing their attention on transforming the city's health department from a preventive to a curative body. No longer would the city respond only in times of epidemics. Instead it would work to provide routine health care. They did this by building programs for public health nursing, housing reform, milk safety, birthing services, and venereal disease treatment and by persuading the city to include these programs in its official infrastructure. As a result, women controlled the daily tasks that safeguarded the public's health, even as men ultimately dominated the top-level positions of authority as health officers and members of boards of health.

Female reformers left a legacy of an expansive municipal public health service. Because of their activities, the health department provided public health nurses to offer home care, physicians to attend to women during childbirth, and clinics for sufferers of venereal disease. Although in many cases these specific programs did not survive past the Great Depression, these women enhanced societal expectations about civic responsibility by bringing health care into working people's homes. Their values and ideas have shaped our modern constructs of what constitutes a public health hazard and its institutional remedy. At the same time, their perceptions of race, class, ethnicity, and gender, as well as their loss of control once they ceded power over their programs to the city health department, limited their progressive stance on public commitments. Still, these women ultimately wanted to make the state, not break it.

Chapter 1

Paid for by the Public Purse
Public Health Nursing

On Monday, November 22, 1897, Los Angeles became the first municipality in the United States to fund a public health nurse.[1] This action answered a petition made six months earlier by Maude B. Foster, president of the Los Angeles College Settlement Association (LACSA).[2] In her request, Foster claimed that the city had already begun taking steps toward acknowledging its responsibility for promoting health. In May 1895, the board of health appointed physician Louise M. Harvey as a sanitary inspector after listening to a report made by LACSA representatives Evelyn Stoddart, Mary Bingham, and Harvey on conditions in "Sonora Town," an immigrant working-class neighborhood in the second ward.[3] The city did not provide pay, however, and limited her authority to the district in question. In the course of her work, Harvey dispensed medical advice and attention. Foster referenced Harvey's activities in her petition to justify LACSA's new request. She argued that LACSA functioned as an important health care center for residents of the city's second ward and that it could no longer shoulder the fiscal burden of caring for the public's health in this district.

Beyond financial considerations, Foster appealed to the city to assert its ideological power over public health. As a Wellesley-educated, affluent, unmarried, socialist woman, Foster believed in the state's capacity for social justice. Neither her biography nor her political philosophy made her exceptional in Los Angeles in this historical period.[4] Foster argued that if the city agreed to fund a nurse, then LACSA would consign a certain degree of control over the program to the city's health department; the city's health officer would select and supervise the nurse in conjunction with LACSA. A brief letter of support from Luther Milton Powers, the city's chief health officer, accompanied LACSA's request.

The city council considered the settlement's petition along with requests from two other local organizations engaged in issues of social welfare, the Boys and Girls Aid Society and the Day Nursery. Initially, the council's finance committee recommended that each group receive a monthly sum of fifteen dollars, an amount not nearly enough for a nurse's salary. The national average was fifty.[5] Lost from the historical record are the documents that would reveal exactly what transpired next, but a process of negotiation must have taken place. Upon councilman Charles H. Toll's recommendation, the city amended the finance committee's suggestion and raised the settlement's appropriation to fifty dollars per month and the other societies' to twenty. While we may never know who or what persuaded Toll to offer this revision, by his action Los Angeles became the first city in the nation to salary a public health nurse.[6]

In return for the funds, the settlement provided the facilities and equipment, and conducted outreach to the city's working poor and the indigent. This joint venture remained publicly financed and privately controlled until the women of LACSA sought and secured the passage of an ordinance to merge the program into the city's health department sixteen years later. By obtaining municipal funding, female reformers in Los Angeles blurred the boundary between private initiative and state responsibility for public health. In developing social services for the city, these women also created a space within which they could direct public policy. Consequently, how they understood germs, motherhood, health, and sickness came to inform the machinery of the local state. Yet reformers' beliefs alone did not structure the distribution of health care in the city. Instead, the negotiations within people's homes among nurses, patients, and their families played a crucial role in shaping the character and expression of LACSA's public health nursing program. As policy makers and as patients, women reconstructed the relationship of the city to its residents.

By establishing a public health nursing program, Los Angeles joined a transatlantic health movement to bring modern medical care into the home.[7] Despite the existence of American charitable organizations in the early nineteenth century that provided home care to the poor, female reformers in the United States in the late nineteenth century looked to England for their model.[8] Yet these programs took on different dimensions in the United States because its health care system was decentralized and localized. In terms of timing, the formation of the Los Angeles program in 1897 was in step with the rest of the country.[9] In terms of civic financing, Los Angeles was in the forefront.

A few years after securing funding from the city, LACSA boasted that it had accomplished in Los Angeles what their counterparts in the East and Midwest could not. They argued that, "no similar request has been considered in Boston, New York, or Chicago."[10] Their observation was truthful in at least one respect: Los Angeles was the only city in the United States to finance a public health nurse in the 1890s. Proud as they were of municipal support, it was not their original plan. Like their counterparts at Hull House, LACSA's leaders initially intended to rely on private philanthropists for the funds to establish and maintain their programs.[11] In an 1897 report, they claimed that garnering the fifty dollars a month for a nurse's salary from local physicians and other interested parties "[did] not seem an impossible accomplishment."[12] Yet that same year LACSA took in just enough funds from its dues and donations to pay for its lease, rent a piano, and purchase the assorted daily necessities for running its already existing programs. The $600 a year they needed for a nurse's salary was more than their entire budget. Their assertion not withstanding, it is reasonable to assume that in addition to a belief about civic responsibility for health, LACSA's leaders turned to the city because there was no one else left to ask.

In their lore, LACSA stressed that the program's origin contrasted sharply from its contemporaries because reformers in other cities had to worry about "the interposition of municipal politics."[13] In making this argument, LACSA perpetuated a stereotype that the standard social geography of city politics inhibited social progress. Because of the absence of a Tammany Hall, LACSA downplayed the existence of partisan politics within Los Angeles. Even so, just a few months before filing their petition, the city council and the board of health were embroiled in a conflict over the power of appointment.[14] Apparently, the employment of C. W. Wright, George Ritzer, Louis Siewiecke, and Edward J. Morris as health inspectors proved "distasteful to the Democratic members of the Council." In late February, the city council passed an ordinance that entitled them to appoint the health department's employees and determine their numbers and salaries.

The board of health and the mayor strenuously objected to this law, arguing that the attenuated supervision would compromise the health of the city. The board of health argued that they had been unfairly singled out. The city council allowed the police, fire, and park departments to maintain complete control over their employees. While a court decision was pending, the council and the board both designated representatives. Consequently, for a period of at least three months two sets of inspectors showed up each day at the health department office. In April, Judge Lucien Shaw reluctantly found in favor of the city council. In examining the city's charter, he determined that the board of health could only make appointments when the city council expressly created ordinances authorizing it to do so. Despite his own finding, he commented "to require [the board of health] to administer the [health] department by means of employees selected by some other body is certainly not tending, in general, to secure the best results." Although LACSA made it seem that political strife over public health did not exist in Los Angeles, given their general attentiveness to city politics and the publicity this particular story received, it is reasonable to conclude that members were aware of this conflict. They might even have used it to their advantage. It is not inconceivable that in the aftermath of these contests the city council funded the nurse to reiterate its ability to control public health appointments.

LACSA's hyperbole extended to declarations about the public health nursing program's unique nature. Although LACSA was the first to receive municipal funds for a nurse, the relationship between public health nursing associations and city health departments was more complicated than LACSA portrayed. Female reformers throughout the nation disagreed over the appropriate connection of nursing programs to official bureaucratic structures. At one end of the spectrum, Mary K. Sedgwick of the Boston Instructive District Nursing Association advised the readers of the *Forum* that "it is most desirable that such work as this shall have no connection with municipal politics, even to the exclusion of the regular city physicians."[15] Private patronage allowed this organization to maintain its independence.

Somewhere in the middle was Lillian D. Wald's arrangement with New York City's health department. Wald originally feared that tenement dwellers would rebuff her attempts to enter, and, consequently, she "desir[ed] to have some connection with civic authority."[16] She sought and secured symbols of coercive power from the city. The president of New York City's board of health granted her badges that proclaimed "Visiting Nurse. Under the Auspices of the Board of Health." In retrospect she said that this turned out to be an unnecessary precaution and in some instances it was not "felicitous to utilize this privilege." At the time, however, Wald did not see the program's association with the board as "a perfunctory or merely complimentary one." Instead, Wald felt that "from the beginning [there was] an inclination on the part of the officials of the department to treat us more or less like comrades." She submitted daily diaries of her work to the district's physician and, in return, "received many encouraging reminders that what we were doing was considered helpful." Working as "comrades," however, did not mean that they received their funds from the same source. Wald relied on voluntary subscriptions to maintain her program. Although Henry Street was famous for distinguishing itself from charity by collecting fees from patients, Wald viewed this as a policy for preserving self-respect rather than expecting that it would generate enough funds to maintain the settlement.

At the other end of the spectrum was LACSA, which would not have been able to execute its nursing program without city funds. In its first three years of existence, LACSA relocated three times and did not establish live-in residents. While members of the settlement movement considered residence a fundamental feature that set their institutions apart from older structures of charity, they argued that LASCA could "probably be welcomed into the circle of settlements" because of its "avowal of an intention to reside."[17]

Although the settlement managed to purchase a permanent home in 1902, it owed this to the philanthropy of one of its members who supplied $1,500 for the down payment. With $2,000 left on the mortgage, the settlement appealed to socially concerned citizens nationwide to fund its endeavor to purchase a permanent home. Apparently this plea did not work because in 1905, the settlement still owed $1,800 on the mortgage.[18] These difficulties raise the question: if they did not have enough money to buy a building, how could they have afforded to pay a nurse's salary? The receipts from the public health nursing program's first nine years of existence reveal that LACSA contributed a very small amount of money in comparison to the city in order to maintain the service. The records indicate that the settlement spent approximately $250 on supplies, while the nurses' salaries came to about $9,500.[19] Patient contributions would have been one means to offset costs, but LACSA instructed its nurses to refuse payment. While they do not explicitly explain the motivation for this rule, accepting funds would have negated its image as a public program. According to the program's guidelines, above all "the nurses [were] public servants" and "after seven years experience, [LACSA was] willing to attest the advantage of a system which supplies nurses for the public, paid from the public purse."[20] Clearly one advantage of this arrangement was that it freed LACSA from diverting funds from its main goal, the permanent security of their settlement house. By refusing payments from patients, however, LACSA opened itself up to accusations of being a charity, a perception that Maude B. Foster lamented "clung" to the settlement movement "like a barnacle."[21]

Securing municipal funds was more than a merely practical solution to the settlement's fiscal problems; it was also philosophically motivated. In 1899, two years after the first municipal appropriation, Foster published an article entitled "The Settlement and Socialism" in the *Commons*.[22] She contended that settlement workers should work "until the causes of poverty are removed, not *ameliorated*" (her emphasis.) While Foster conceded that settlement workers often created kindergartens, public bathhouses, and libraries to "protest against existing municipal conditions," she also asked "but is [this work] not equally a menace to municipal interest?" She went on to argue that "the municipality's function has been disregarded, ignored, and minimized." According to Foster, if settlements permanently privatized what she believed to be public services, then they would be making a fundamental mistake in their reform efforts. Thus, from her socialist perspective, Los Angeles's municipal government had taken a major step toward fulfilling its proper role by paying the salary of the public health nurse. Given the popularity of socialism in Los Angeles during this period, she could have reasonably concluded that her opinion would find favor.[23] Foster's political perspective also helps to explain why she eventually agitated to have the city formally incorporate public health nursing into its official public health infrastructure.

LACSA's difficulty in securing financing for a nurse are reminders of the ambivalent attitude held by many toward the settlement movement. Yet LACSA's use of public funds to support its nursing program made it vulnerable to a distinctly different type of public censure than elsewhere. Citizens could petition the city government to exercise control over the public purse, and they did. While Foster encouraged the municipal government in Los Angeles to adopt settlement-inspired programs, other local residents demanded that the city council step in and quash the experiment. A group of business owners, skilled and semiskilled workers, and other assorted neighboring residents petitioned the city in 1899 and 1901 to take action against the settlement.[24] They had two complaints. In 1899, they claimed that LACSA was a public nuisance. In 1901, they argued that financing the nurse was an illegitimate use of public money. Both the settlement and its critics advocated government action on behalf of the city's residents, but they disagreed over defining whose welfare was at risk and how it could be protected.

Edward Bouton and Herman Zuber led the fight against the settlement both times. Bouton was a retired brigadier general, president of the Bouton Water Company and the Capistrano Oil Company, and a resident of the area for twenty-seven years. Zuber owned a truck and transfer company. Thirteen men and women, but mostly men, signed the petition in 1899 and seventeen in 1901. Of these, only four were repeats. The range of surnames—Dutch, English, French, Irish, Italian, German, Polish, Scottish, Scotch-Irish, and Spanish—suggest that the protest was not limited by ethnicity. Judging by the city directories, a number of petitioners were small-business owners (peddler, baker, boardinghouse keeper, saloon keeper, and grocer) and others were skilled and semiskilled workers (mason, car cleaner, wheelwright, pressman, engineer, conductor, grader, and hostler). The majority of petitioners owned their homes. Zuber lived next door to the settlement and Bouton's residence was cater corner from it. Most of the other petitioners lived on the same block as the settlement or within walking distance. The battle over the settlement's presence in this mixed-class residential neighborhood spoke to the tensions wrought by late-nineteenth-century urbanism. In addition, these fights would not have occurred unless the settlement had secured some measure of success with the working-class people who came to it.

In 1899, the petitioners asserted that they were acting to protect their families, neighborhood, and property from "the boys" who visited the settlement. Their wanton behavior consisted of "occupying the streets, indulging in various games, wrestling, fighting, swearing and using the most vulgar and obscene language, pilfering, pillaging, and throwing stones into adjacent premises." The petitioners found it offensive that "all passer[s]-by [were] compelled to hear the most vulgar and profane utterances imaginable." In 1901, the accusations went beyond the use of indecent language to purported predatory behavior. In an affidavit attached to the petition, Mrs. E. Pierret charged the boys with sexual assault. She insisted that a little girl "who was then living at my house . . . was just going into the College Settlement Building to get a library book, when she was seized, thrown down off the porch, her clothes thrown up, and she was roughly handled." Older girls heard her screams and came to her aid. Pierret blamed the "College Settlement Gang" and stated that despite her protestations, Foster did not take any action.

The city council responded to each petition by turning the matter over to committee for investigation.[25] In each case, the settlement did not dispute the boys' crude behavior. One of the settlement's founders, Evelyn Stoddart, "admitted that the boys swear, but said they are not now as profane as formerly." Stoddart did not concede, however, that the boys who visited the settlement were the perpetrators of the physical assault.

It became apparent in the course of these inquiries that the initial source of turbulence stemmed from a skirmish over the use of private space for public leisure. Zuber and Bouton had obstructed the boys' baseball games when they developed two vacant lots in the area. They plowed one up and placed "a large machine" with one wheel removed "so that it could not be taken out of the way" on the other. The boys retaliated by contesting the rules of decorum. Not only did they swear but at one point on their way to LACSA's bathhouse they "stripped stark naked, and in a nude condition, paraded over the top of the bath-house, roof, and about the premises." Bouton and Zuber apparently had "tried to drive the boys away by the use of whips." The boys responded by destroying Bouton's "hedges, fences and trees." It was within the context of these continuing clashes between men and boys over public space that the public health nurse came under attack.

Despite the rhetoric of the 1899 petition, it was limited in its demands. The petitioners wanted to be rid of the "intolerable nuisance," but they knew that the city lacked the power to evict LACSA from the neighborhood. Consequently, they asked for a policeman to "be permanently stationed on [the] corner [of Alpine and Castelar] to maintain order and keep these boys under restraint." The city rejected their request. Moreover, the city council found "that the College Settlement [was] an influence, not for evil, but for good, and that it deserve[d] much more general support from the public than it ha[d] hitherto received." The council highlighted the presence of the nurse as a positive influence.

Three years later, the petitioners tried again but this time they mounted an offensive specifically against the nurse. They began their petition by asserting their rights as "tax-payers" to influence the public purse. They expressed exasperation that their money was helping to "sustain an institution that owing to the very peculiar, and, as [they thought] erroneous and utterly impractical theories of the managers . . . [was] doing a great deal of harm." The petitioners contended that their community did not need this form of public assistance and objected to the stigma it carried. They questioned LACSA's assertion that the second ward was a locus for disease: "Since the founding of the Pueblo, that section has been noted as the most healthy portion of the city, and there is less need of the services of a nurse there than in any other locality." Although they did not deny that some poorer residents lived in the area, they disputed the belief that the majority needed help from the state: "The people residing in that section are generally industrious, thrifty, and prosperous, and the number that are not able to pay for the services of a nurse, should they require one, is very small indeed." The articulation of these demands suggests they did not completely contest the idea that the city could provide health care for its poorer residents. Instead, they rejected its application in this particular locale.

In defense of the nurse, the settlement called Jose Franco, who lived next door to Zuber, to testify. Franco claimed that the "boys [did] not bother him and would not Gen. Bouton and Mr. Zuber if they did not nag them." He argued that the "work of the nurse in the section is of great good and the residents regard the College Settlement as a protection and a refuge." LACSA also called Oscar Chavez, a former neighborhood "boy," to speak about the settlement's impact on his life. He testified that the "reason he could make a speech to the Councilmen [was] because he learned much at the Settlement that [was] beneficial and helpful. . . . To these ladies . . . I owe all that I know about parliamentary law and official procedure." He also stated that the nurse was "doing much good. This very day I have a case to report where a woman is lying sick in bed unattended. She has six little children and no means. I shall tell the ladies of the College Settlement Association and I know that the woman will have the best of care. She will not be left to the unsympathetic attention of the general medical authorities." Franco's comments suggest a general distrust of the health department from which LACSA's nurse appears to have been exempt. In this case, as in the last, the city council sided with the settlement, and a week later it disbursed its annual allocation to LACSA for its nurse.[26]

Although unsuccessful, the attack on the nurse demonstrates that not all of the public agreed with the city council's decision to create this quasi-public program. Moreover, the program's public status made it vulnerable to civic protest in ways quite different from other public health nursing associations across the country. At the same time, the creation of this program within a female-dominated institution resembled the work being done in Boston and New York. In these ways, the Los Angeles program was unique but not exceptional within the context of social and urban reform taking place during this historical period. By focusing our attention on the development and maintenance of the program itself, we can see the other ways in which the settlement trod contested terrain. Above all, LACSA challenged the city to redefine its role in relationship to the health of its residents.

During the sixteen years under the College Settlement's supervision, the public health nurses took care of 21,749 patients and made 102,446 visits to people's homes. The nurses most commonly saw patients for what they termed "unclassified" diseases: colds, sores, and minor infections. "Febrile and zymotic diseases" constituted the second most numerous type of health problem the nurses attended to in their work. "Febrile" referred to fever-producing symptoms and "zymotic" to the process of fermentation. Scientists, physicians, and public health officials used the term "zymotic" to describe diseases whose origin they believed lay in filth, were contagious, and transmitted through the air. These terms were still frequently used during the early years in which scientists determined that bacterial agents caused disease. As historians have demonstrated, the germ theory did not immediately revolutionize either the public's understanding of disease nor physicians' practices.[27] The Los Angeles city health department used "zymotic" in the 1890s but had abandoned the term in favor of "infectious diseases" by 1904.[28] LACSA never updated its taxonomy. Without any direct commentary by LACSA on its methods for categorizing disease, it is difficult to draw conclusions about its decision to retain its original classification system.

Foster did not permit the nurses to "diagnose or prescribe for a case" because she believed this work more properly belonged "to the physician." Instead, she charged the nurses with being able to recognize a "gamut of diseases," including typhoid fever, tuberculosis, diphtheria, influenza, measles, whooping cough, mumps, and smallpox, that regularly affected their patients. Recognition stemmed from experience, not a laboratory finding.[29] Moreover, LACSA's focus on environmental remedies remained the same whether the prevailing theory on the origin of disease specified the source as filth or germs. Consequently, from the perspective of LACSA it might have been less important what specific taxonomy was used to classify the diseases the nurses encountered than recording the numbers of patients that they were treating.

The location of immigrant communities essentially predetermined the geographic parameters of the association's nursing program because surveys of neighborhood conditions and muckracking exposés from across the nation posited a relationship between rates of disease and immigrant working-class neighborhoods.[30] One of the first activities LASCA undertook was to conduct an investigation of sanitary conditions in its immediate vicinity. Although public health nurses worked primarily in the "field," the settlement functioned as their headquarters. The Los Angeles College Settlement was located at the southeast corner of Alpine and Castelar, northwest of the Plaza, in what would now be considered Chinatown just north of downtown. The nurses traveled most often in the immediate vicinity of the settlement but also extended their work southward along both sides of the Los Angeles River. In total, the settlement identified a territory 2½ miles to 3 miles in length and a mile wide as its primary concern. In 1900, over 40,000 people lived within this area, 49 percent of whom were foreign born.[31]

Although LACSA argued that "the immigrant problem in our midst is a diversified picture," the settlement's qualitative descriptions of patient-nurse interaction concentrated on Mexicans and Russians.[32] Settlement workers' beliefs about who would be most and least receptive to their prescriptions for health contributed to their focus on these two ethnic groups. According to LACSA, Mexicans were gullible and affable and Russians were aggressively stubborn and superstitious. These opinions were not always borne out by the nurses' experiences nor did these characterizations remain static, yet they played an important role in guiding the settlement's work.[33]

Mexicans always composed the largest percentage of the nurses' patients throughout the association's history and, consequently, were their focus. There were demographic reasons for this emphasis. "American" patients decreased from 14 percent of the nurses' clientele in 1898 to just 3 percent by the time the association amalgamated its program into the city's health department in 1913. Italians and Russians decreased from their rolls in similar proportions (Italians 13 percent to 4 percent, Russians from 6 percent to 1 percent).

Mexicans, however, increased from 49 percent to 83 percent of the nurses' patients. One reason for these statistics was that the settlement had located in an area where Mexicans were forced to live as others moved out; residential segregation limited Mexican mobility. In addition, the Mexican Revolution led to an increase in the overall numbers of Mexicans living within the city.[34] Thus, LACSA's statistics reflected changes in residential-living patterns that were affected by early-twentieth-century racial dynamics and geopolitics.

Studying LACSA's public health nursing program provides insights into how settlement workers collaborated with city government in an attempt to make the "city livable."[35] Although this relationship was not without tension, it stands in contrast to the experience of female reformers in other cities because the municipality remained committed to paying the nurses' salaries. In the sixteen years following its initial appropriation, the city council allocated money for four more nurses, bringing the total number up to five who worked under LACSA's supervision. The city council also raised the nurses' salaries from fifty to seventy-five dollars a month plus carfare.[36] The city council records provide little detail as to why they acquiesced so amenably to LACSA's requests. One reasonable explanation is the personal connections that existed between the public health nursing program's manager, Maude Foster, and members of the Los Angeles business community.

Maude Foster Weston was the chief architect of LACSA's public health nursing program.[37] Scholars have analyzed middle-class and elite women's motivations and engagement in reform efforts at the turn of the twentieth century, and much of Weston's story sounds typical: affluent upbringing, college educated, and single when she began working in reform (Maude Foster married pianist Nathan Weston in Los Angeles in 1902).[38] Like the experiences of many other settlement workers, Weston's ability to engage in reform was made possible by inherited wealth and a family support network, especially help from her twin sister, Nancy Foster.

Weston was born in 1865 in Pittsburgh to a wealthy family. Her father was a coal merchant in the steel capital of the world. According to the United States Census Manuscript of 1870, John W. Foster's total worth was valued at $30,000, the relative worth of which was approximately a half-million dollars in 2007.[39] In sharing his life history with the Los Angeles Public Library, Weston's older brother Ernest K. Foster noted that his mother, Mary Elizabeth Kidd Foster, died in August 1866. With three young children, the twins just over a year old, their father remarried between 1866 and 1870. His second wife, Bella Foster, subsequently bore two children, John and Anna. In August 1871, John W. Foster died, leaving a pregnant wife and four children. Nonetheless, the family stayed financially solvent. The census manuscript from 1880 indicates that all five children were attending school and that the family was able to hire a cook, a chambermaid, and a servant to attend to their needs.

Ernest K. Foster pioneered the family's migration to Los Angeles. In the midst of a real estate boom, he moved to the city in 1886 and set up shop as a commercial printer and engraver. He later became an investment banker and served as a director of the Los Angeles Public Library before ill health claimed his life in 1927. Ernest's wife, Caroline Holcomb Wright Foster, was born in Greenfield, Ohio, and moved to Los Angeles in 1889. She was a writer, a charter member of the Friday Morning Club, and a founder of the local Juvenile Protection Association, and she served as president of the first Board of Motion Picture Census. Maude and Nancy Foster joined their older brother in Los Angeles in 1894. Four years later, John Foster also joined the family there. According to William A. Spalding, John D. Foster was a "real estate man" and "a prominent figure in civic affairs, being an ardent supporter of every movement which had as its object the well-being of society and gave freely of his time and means to those ends." John married Kathleen Acheson, who became a founding member of the Los Angeles Country Club and was "a member of a number of civic organizations and [had] always been identified with movements for the betterment of the community." Anna Foster joined her siblings sometime between 1905 and 1910. She arrived with her husband, Samuel F. Hammond, and two young sons.[40]

The presence of the Foster family enabled Weston to engage in social reform. First, she was not the only member of the family to participate in the settlement movement. Caroline was present at the opening of the settlement in 1895 and reportedly one of its first "workers."[41] In 1896, Nancy lectured on *Don Quixote* at the settlement's La Primavera Club, which she also helped run.[42] In addition, the First Instructive District Nursing Report listed Anna as one of the two women in charge of the Uniforms and Supply Stations committee. Altruistic activities combined with family finances. The Foster family collectively contributed 17 percent of the total private funding the settlement received from 1894 to 1897. Weston's donation of sixty-eight dollars and eighty cents made her the second-highest single contributor.[43] In these ways this story sounds similar to Hull House, where Addams successfully parlayed personal relationships into investments. Unfortunately, further documentation does not exist to track LACSA's fund-raising efforts or its fiscal contributors. Still, although speculative, it is not unreasonable to conclude that these interpersonal relationships fostered Weston's ability to favorably influence civic leaders.

In addition to family connections, Weston also belonged to another network: college alumnae. When she was eighteen, Weston and her identical twin sister enrolled at Wellesley College as "special students." Wellesley devised this category for women who wished to take classes but not matriculate into a particular program and receive a degree. In the two years that Weston attended, 1883 to 1884, "specials" accounted for over a third of the school's total enrollment. Wellesley stipulated that "specials" be at least eighteen, in good health, present character references, and be able to keep up in the regular classes. According to her transcript, Weston selected courses in chemistry, botany, logic, literature, French, Bible study, and elocution.[44] While Weston did not obtain formal training as a nurse, which contrasted with Lillian Wald's experience, her studies imbued her with a sense of scientific methodology and morality. These, she believed, were the crucial elements of public health nursing. In sum, Weston can be viewed as a combination of what contemporaries labeled as a "lady manager" with what would soon be called a "new woman."[45] She may not have been a nurse but she was college educated and of a professionalizing generation.[46] Settlement work offered an enticing vocational outlet to this generation in transition.

Where Weston and her sister were between their time at Wellesley and moving to Los Angeles is unclear. Maude paid at least one visit to the city in 1889, where reports of her excursions made the society column of the *Los Angeles Times*.[47] Judging by the city directories, the sisters permanently moved to the city in 1894 when they were twenty-nine. After residing for a few months in the Hotel Figueroa, a YWCA facility, they purchased a house at 643 West 32nd Street, where they lived until their deaths in the 1940s. Hence, they moved to southern California in the same year in which the Los Angeles branch of the National Association of Collegiate Alumnae established its settlement. Weston's Wellesley connection mattered because at least three of the founding members of LACSA were Wellesley alumnae.[48] The settlement's newness and uncertain future provided Weston with opportunities. Her active participation led her to the position of secretary in 1896 and president the following year. During her tenure in the latter position, the settlement persuaded the city to provide the funds with which LACSA could hire a public health nurse.

With municipal funding in place, Weston supervised the activities of the nurse, Miss McRae, who lived in residence at the settlement.[49] At the end of 1908, when the program grew to include three nurses, Weston began publishing a formal report of its activities. She printed a set of rules at the end of the report, and it was through these rules that Weston formed the character of the Instructive District Nursing Association for the City of Los Angeles. They codified the different attributes that made public health nursing a distinct profession. These rules also helped institutionalize the program's place within the city's public health infrastructure.

Weston's "Rules for Nurses" set forth decrees on hours, salary, uniforms, and equipment. Unless responding to an emergency, the nurses worked between the hours of 8:30 A.M. and 5:00 P.M., Monday through Saturday. The nurses had a right to one month's vacation, without salary, and could take two personal half-days each month. These stipulations assured the public health nurse greater potential for autonomy than her private-duty counterpart. Despite national disagreement among the leaders of the public health nursing movement about the wearing of uniforms—some feared it bore too close a resemblance to the frocks of religious orders—Weston chose to make uniforms a requirement. Wearing the required blue-and-white uniform symbolized the nurses' professional status as well as advertised their presence in the city.[50] She also required the nurses to equip themselves with an "inexpensive watch and a fountain pen." Obliging the nurses to keep time and write daily reports turned these items into symbolic accoutrements of professionalization.

The rules also defined what qualified as appropriate types of work. According to Weston, the three tenets of public health nursing were discovery,

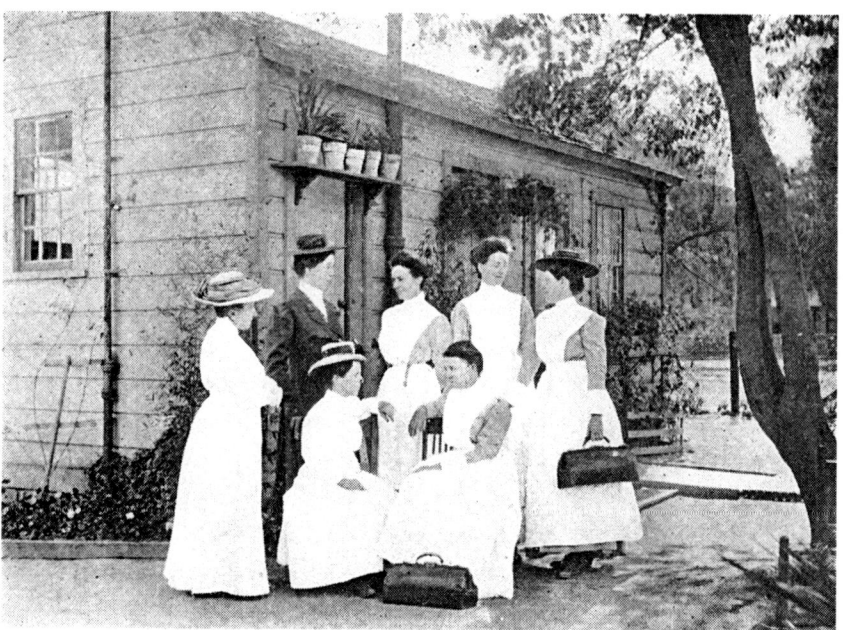

Figure 1 Maude Foster Weston and the public health nurses struck poses evocative of their professionalism.

(Source: The College Settlement, *The Twelfth Report of Instructive District Nursing for the City of Los Angeles under the Supervision of the College Settlement* [1908–1910], History and Special Collections Division, Louise M. Darling, Biomedical Library, UCLA)

instruction, and prevention. Weston expected the nurses to investigate the family's health and their environmental surroundings. She required the nurses to sanitize the "sick-room," which in reality often meant attending to the patient's entire home. Weston also viewed the nurses as the city's alarm system, reporting any immediate health dangers to the proper authorities. This made the nurses mediators between physicians and patients and between city support services, residents, and organized charities.

Yet, while Weston envisioned the purview of public health nursing as quite broad, she did specify certain limits. For instance, Weston forbade nurses from "visiting in houses of prostitution." If LACSA's goal was to "help the privileged and the unprivileged to a better understanding of their mutual obligations," then Weston was not going to enter into a partnership with sex workers.[51] She also prohibited nurses from working with midwives. Midwives symbolized folk traditions to Weston that she believed were incompatible with the presence of modern medicine as symbolized by the nurse (see chapter 4). Most importantly, although she viewed her nurses as using scientific methods for investigation and treatment, she believed that physicians possessed a different and greater medical authority. Consequently, Weston barred nurses from acting as substitute doctors. "Professional etiquette," she declared, "demands that in their work for physicians, the nurses are not allowed to diagnose nor prescribe for any case."[52] Acting in such a manner would have superseded their authority and hence negated their legitimacy as professionals. Sometimes, however, physicians proved uncooperative in acknowledging this partnership. Weston recounted an instance where "an irresponsible doctor, in response to my insisting upon better care of a young mother replied: 'If you do not stop interfering with my case, I'll have you arrested.'"[53] Undaunted, Weston argued that "we are not in the field to criticize unjustly, but we are there to save life. And we mean to do it." Through these policies, Weston sought to carve out a distinct professional space for the public health nurse and as such "no society or doctor ha[d] any special claim upon their time."[54]

According to Weston, those who did have a claim to the public health nurses were the "sick poor of Los Angeles."[55] In practical terms, this meant the immigrant working-class population who lived in close proximity to the settlement. Consequently, Weston found herself managing not only class conflicts between the region's neighbors and interactions between physicians and nurses but also interethnic interactions between the nurses and their patients.

Public health officials and LACSA's settlement workers sought to deal with current-day realities, but narratives about the region's history and perceptions of immigrant health customs influenced the construction of their programs.

Weston, for instance, specifically distinguished Mexicans from Californios (allegedly descendants of Spanish colonists) upon whom romantic visions and portrayals, such as *Ramona*, had been built.[56] Weston argued that "to many of us, the Mexican seems to belong to California, but it is not the descendants of the early Californians that we find in the courtyards, and who are the majority of our patients," instead "it is the Mexican peon who comes over the border to build our railroads, he who lives in the 'construction camps.' "[57] Weston stated, "We may not like him nor his habits or customs, but he is in our midst—he is omnipresent." The problem from a public health perspective was the reliance of Mexican immigrants on folk medicine. She believed that Mexicans had a "natural tendency to believe in the 'Medicine-man' and the 'Curendera,' and is an easy prey to this sort of doctoring, especially is this the case among the pregnant women."[58] In speaking to a crowd of reform-minded men and women in March 1898, a few months after the city's initial allocation of funds, Weston argued that the primary importance of hiring a nurse was to "save the people from irregular practitioners, or in other words quackery."[59]

In describing LACSA's program at a conference of social workers held in Los Angeles in 1912, Weston maintained that immigrant Russians caused the nurses the greatest trouble in carrying out their work. She described them as being "full of superstition" and suggested that this mind-set led them to adopt a "fatalistic attitude towards the sick."[60] "To be told that 'the Evil Spirit is upon him' when a patient is burning with fever," she said, "is rather disheartening even to the most courageous nurse." Consequently, Weston believed that Russian attitudes toward disease created "the greatest possible hindrance in our efforts to help them." The solution, according to Weston, was education.

By Weston's logic, immigrants would forsake folk medicine if they learned about the virtues of cleanliness. Although the nursing reports are silent as to how Weston and the nurses understood the advent of the germ theory in relation to their work, the absence of a discussion suggests the flexibility of sanitation. Whether one believed that dirt or microbes caused disease, hygienic practices often responded to both concerns. Weston "held" the nurses "responsible for the condition of the patients when sending them to hospitals, and for the cleanliness of the sick-room." She also officially charged the nurses with "instruct[ing] the family in all such service as well as in the special care of the case." The nurses' reports indicate that they followed through on Weston's orders. They often discussed the ministrations they gave to patients' bodies and the environment within which patients lived. For instance, while waiting for a physician to arrive to treat, "Mrs. B.," "a young Mexican woman" who appeared to be suffering from pneumonia, the nurse "gave [her] a bath and cleaned the bed and room."

Similarly, in attending to "Mrs. M., a tuberculous [sic] case," the nurse "gave baths, alcohol rubs, dressed bedsores, and cleaned room and bed," and "also prepared food." Where possible, the nurses asked family members to maintain the hygienic atmosphere they had established as best they could.[61]

Teaching about the relationship between sanitation and disease might have proved difficult for the nurses because they did not generally speak the same language as their patients. In managing interethnic relations, Weston appears to have diverged from the strategy adopted by other nursing associations of hiring ethnic nurses to aid in issues of translation. Instead, she did not require the nurses to be multilingual. She described the "knowledge of foreign tongues" as "an asset" but "not a chief requirement; for after a very short time among our foreign population, each nurse learns a little 'clinical Spanish,' which is the foreign tongue most needed in Los Angeles."[62] While few documents from LACSA's nurses attest to the problems this posed, a contemporary in Nanticoke, Pennsylvania, conveyed what perhaps these nurses might have felt. In aiding state officials in coping with a typhoid epidemic, Alice M. Halloran wrote to a friend and fellow nurse about the difficulties she experienced due to language barriers: "The inhabitants are mostly foreigners, Polish, Hungarians, & Italians (When I leave I expect to be a Linguist), this makes the situation a difficult one to handle."[63]

Beyond managing ethnic encounters, Weston also attempted to manage gender dynamics. Although the association worked with entire families, Weston emphasized to her staff that they should focus on the needs of women and children. According to Weston and the nurses, Mexican women proved to be the most amenable to their sympathetic and scientific approach for promoting health. Weston wrote, "The Mexican woman is glad to make the little garments, when the material is given, and is apt in following the nurse's instructions."[64] In one particular case where a nurse treated an infant with "gonorrhea opthalmia," which prevented the child from being placed within a hospital, the nurse recounted how the Mexican mother and grandmother were "quick to grasp the instructions given and the necessity of prompt attention and the disposal of the infected dressings." According to the nurse's report, the women had been "very grateful" to her "for the assistance given." Despite these positive experiences, Weston considered Mexican and Russian ethnicity as potential limits to the bonds of womanhood. She felt that Mexicans displayed a propensity toward gullibility and Russians toward obstinacy that interfered with the association's public health work.

Weston selected who would work in the program. This meant that although the nurses were in Weston's words "public servants," they did not have the protections of civil servants. Instead, they were always subject to Weston's assessment as to their worthiness. Weston judged her nurses' characters against those valued by Florence Nightingale. In an address before a conference of social workers that was held in May 1912 in Los Angeles, Weston stated: "Florence Nightingale, the forerunner of all trained nurses, placed her seal upon what I consider some of the essential requirements. She was a gentlewoman, a woman of intellect, and a Christian woman of force and ability."[65] Using these criteria, Weston fired one nurse "for the manner in which she threw off the sheet on the bed of a poor tuberculosis woman" and another because she "lacked enduring quality." As Susan Reverby has stated, nurses were "ordered to care."[66]

Yet, although Weston argued, "the best women I have had on the staff have never been wholly of a 'professional' type," she preferred to hire graduates from certified nursing programs.[67] She expressed frustration that she had to spend too much time convincing the "lone widow" and "capable masseuse" that they were unsuited for the job.[68] These were traditional points of entry into practical nursing, but Weston disqualified these sorts of women because they lacked diplomas. Weston believed that specialized schooling endowed public health nurses with a "modern and scientific manner." Intuition helped in treating diseases but not in identifying their causes; leaders of public health nursing asserted that searching for "the cause" set public health nursing apart within the profession. Although she was not trained in nursing herself, Weston's blending of sympathy and science in defining the key elements of public health nursing was in alignment with that espoused by leaders in the movement to professionalize nursing and social work.

Weston employed fourteen nurses during her sixteen years as supervisor. All those listed in the annual reports had, without exception, obtained some hospital training. Although the majority received their education in the East, Weston did not limit her hiring from any particular hospital. Most of the nurses attained their training in cities (New York and Buffalo; Lowell, Lynn, and Fall River in Massachusetts) that were among the fifty most populous from 1890 to 1910. Only two nurses received their primary training in California, one at the Cottage Hospital in Santa Barbara and the other at the Los Angeles County Hospital.

Using the 1920 and 1930 censuses we can discover a little bit more about eight of these nurses. All of them were what the U.S. Census categorized as "white." Two were foreign born, one from England and the other from Canada. Their average age when they began working at the settlement was thirty-two. In 1930, almost all were unmarried. Five of these eight women were living with their sisters. Judging by their last names, these women also tended to have remained single. They worked in jobs that we would now consider pink collar. In only one case was someone's sister also listed as a nurse; the other occupations enumerated included teachers and stenographers. The 1930 Census manuscript provided an estimated value for houses and rents, and it indicates that five out of the eight women owned their own homes in 1930. The mean value of these homes was $7,000.[69] Putting together these bits of evidence, it is reasonable to assert that these women occupied what might be considered a gray area between being members of the middle class and working class in the early twentieth century. The word "middling" perhaps better suits as a description. In comparison, Weston and her sister also owned their own home, which was valued at $18,000 in 1930. Interestingly, they had also remained together throughout their lives (Weston's husband moved into her house). In sum, the census data highlight some similarities between the nurses and their manager: both managed to obtain a certain degree of social and economic independence in an era when most women's lives followed a different trajectory. These data, however, also indicate the heterogeneity of experience within the middle class of the early twentieth century.

Weston included several pages of nurses' records in the twelfth annual report (1908–1910), which she claimed to have left unaltered. While the report is still a problematic source for uncovering the voices of the nurses—for instance, it does not provide any negative commentary from the nurses about the management of the program—in the absence of more direct archival material it does provide some clues about the experience of the nurses working in the program. The texts suggest how the nurses viewed their relationship with those who used their services and their belief in the importance of their role in helping to take care of the public's health. They document a record of helping patients to manage medical care: dressing and redressing of wounds, explaining how to administer medication, and creating a therapeutic environment for recovery. Some recounted routine encounters, others focused on emergency situations. The following example is one of the latter.

According to one nurse's record, the settlement received a call from a physician working for the health department asking for immediate assistance at a residence. (The city health department hired physicians to respond to calls of possible contagious disease.) The settlement sent a nurse to the location, where she found a family of Russian Jews "panic-stricken, unable to explain anything." A fifteen-year-old male led her to the kitchen, where she saw an eight-year-old boy lying on the floor surrounded by three physicians. The nurse recalled: "With a word of recognition from the doctors I began to assist them." She deduced by the "loud labored respirations, that this was a case of diphtheria."

The physicians inserted a tube to aid the boy's breathing and decided after a "hurried consultation" between themselves and the family to send the child to the county hospital. At this point the physicians departed and the nurse was "left alone with the patient" until the ambulance came.

According to the nurse, however, this was not a time of relaxation. Instead her patient "needed constant attention" because "mucus accumulating in the throat had to be wiped away, and the cloths burned." In addition, his "coughing was frequent" and at one moment "suddenly, with a convulsive jerk, the tube was coughed up!" The result was that the "pulse became weak, the patient cyanosed, and was collapsing quickly." Although she recognized that her patient would die if the tube were not reinserted, the nurse did not have the medical training to reinsert it, nor did she try. Yet she still had to work to save her patient. She called to the family to run and get "the family physician, who lived very near at hand, or the first physician they could get a hold of and rush to the house." Then she proceeded to give the boy a shot of strychnine, placed

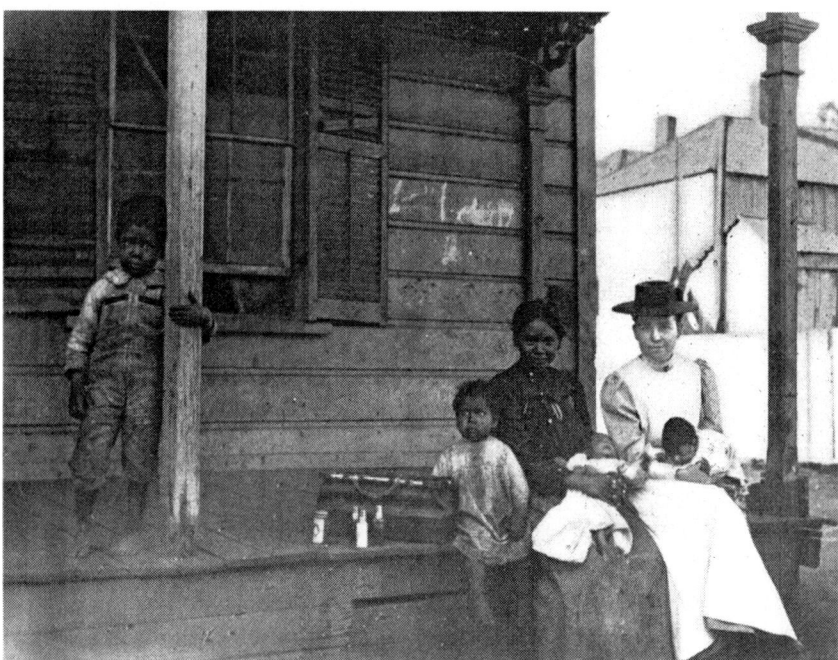

Figure 2 Originally entitled "A Friendly Visit," public health nurses worked to bring municipal health care into people's homes.

(Source: The College Settlement, *The Twelfth Report of Instructive District Nursing for the City of Los Angeles under the Supervision of the College Settlement* [1908–1910], History and Special Collections Division, Louise M. Darling, Biomedical Library, UCLA)

"hot applications" to the boy's "extremities," and then tried a hypodermic stimulant. However he "was sinking fast" so she "gave artificial respiration until arrival of physicians." Once a physician was there, the tube was replaced and the physician stayed. Shortly thereafter the ambulance arrived and the physician accompanied the child to the hospital. The nurse completed her report by indicating that the boy "made a good recovery."

The story suggests how public health nurses represented the city and advocated for the family. Although the rules limited their actions, their activities were still quite broad. In working to save this boy's life, the nurse executed independent judgment both in her attempts at resuscitation and in calling for help. She mediated the relationship between the family and the physicians and the relationship between medical diagnostics and treatment. Furthermore, she utilized both science and sympathy to assert her authority. While Weston dictated the rules regulating this behavior, it was the nurse who controlled her own workspace while in the field. The majority of the nurse's reports included in Weston's twelfth annual report suggest the success in the nurses's ability to garner cooperation among their patients. In this emergency situation, for instance, it appears that contests over treatment were muted. This was not always the case.

What did it mean to the public who availed themselves of LACSA's program to have the city pay for these services? For one thing, the entrance of the public health nurse turned private homes into objects of state inspection. Nurses made door-to-door visits looking for people to help and diseases to report. Thus, they functioned as a means of surveillance. At the same time, however, the nurse was not always uninvited, and the records left by the nurses suggest that patients participated in shaping LACSA's program. As with the nurses, the patients did not leave archival records in their own voice; instead, we need to read between the lines of the official records to extrapolate this evidence. What LACSA's records suggest is that the public health nurse and the public engaged in a process of negotiation in determining the course of health care that was given and received. What is also clear from these documents is that those who interacted with LACSA's public health nurses desired access to medical services even when they disagreed with the ways the nurses wanted to implement care.

What was this process of negotiation? The opening vignette to this book of the thirty-five-year-old Russian woman who had recently given birth but was making a slow recovery demonstrates the ways in which families interceded in determining medical care. The nurse did not attempt to compel the woman to go to the hospital, which was her inclination, because of the family's objections. While the nurse bent to the family's will on this point, she would not accommodate their reticence in giving medications. The nurse coerced the family into acquiescence on this issue by threatening to withhold care.

Similar attempts at intimidation did not necessarily have the same effect. In calling upon "Mrs. W.," who had given birth in the past forty-eight hours, the nurse found that the new mother had been deserted by her husband three months prior and had since been moving with her two-year-old son from friend to friend as long as they could lodge her.[70] The nurse wanted to wash and clean Mrs. W. to prevent infection but found that the woman "obstinately refused" these ministrations "until told she would be reported to a policeman and taken to the hospital." Afterwards, the nurse also wanted to make the bed but encountered further resistance because Mrs. W. would not allow the two-year-old to be removed from her side and the nurse could not remake the bed with both of them in it. The nurse believed that Mrs. W. refused this aid because she "fear[ed] that he would be taken away from her." The nurse did not acknowledge her miscalculation in the negotiations. Instead, she argued that Mrs. W. seemed "very fond of this boy, but did not seem to love the little baby as well." She supported her contention by noting that in a follow-up visit five days later, Mrs. W. had left the newborn with "the woman she was living with, knowing this woman would feed it, having been recently confined," and took her two-year-old with her to visit neighbors. Adding insult to injury, Mrs. W. also refused to eat food brought by the Associated Charities, choosing instead to "live on crackers and milk." Mrs. W. seemed unwilling to conform to the public health nurse's expectations and, consequently, the nurse decided to inform the Humane Society.[71] If we read this story from a slightly different angle, we can say that Mrs. W. felt well enough to get out of bed and had joined forces with another single mother to cope with the problems of child care.

The nurses' reports record the existence of a number of female support networks within working-class communities, although they are not singled out as such. The record related to "Mrs. H." is a case in point. The nurse found Mrs. H. living in a small room in the rear of another woman's house, which she described as "an old shack." Abandoned by her husband three months before, Mrs. H. had just given birth. The nurse expressed concern about the lack of windows in the room and the substitution of "a bundle of dirty rags" for a mattress. The nurse insisted that these circumstances posed a danger to Mrs. H.'s health in her time of confinement so the woman gave Mrs. H. her own room and bed. The nurse did not characterize the other woman's relationship to Mrs. H., making it impossible to assess her acts as motivated by kindness, obligation, or a combination. Prior to giving birth, Mrs. H. had supported herself and her two children by shelling nuts. In returning to that work two weeks later, she left the newborn with the woman while taking the two toddlers with her. In another case, Mrs. G., a mother of five, was able to live with the godmother of one of her children after her husband left her. The woman had come to the nurse's attention after having given birth to twins. The nurse asked the woman how she was planning to support herself, to which the woman replied that with some help she could arrange to leave the city and move to her sister-in-law's ranch. The nurse reported the case to the Associated Charities, who eventually assisted in facilitating the move. While the nurses recounted story after story of desertion, presumably to persuade an audience other than their patients as to the worthiness of their work, they also detail how women turned to other women for places to live and for child care in order to survive.

Recent mothers were not the only people who used the nurses' aid. The reports included one case where a patient called on the nurses instead of the reverse. LACSA kept a station open at the settlement for drop-in visits. "Mr. O." appeared the day after he had cut his arm open with a saw. He had treated the gash with coal oil and black pepper. When the nurse removed the bandage she saw an "angry looking wound." The nurse did not cast aspersions onto Mr. O.'s home remedy, instead choosing to focus on describing her own work in making a blister to cover the area, washing it, and applying an antiseptic solution. She stated that she redressed the wound three times, after which she felt it was sufficiently on the mend and Mr. O. could take care of it himself.

While there are not enough cases in the annual reports to make a definitive determination about the relationship between the type of health care being requested and the degree of acquiescence, these various cases do suggest that childbirth and accidents elicited different responses. While Mr. O. solicited help for his wound, Mrs. W., Mrs. H., and Mrs. G. do not appear to have sought out the nurse. Instead, it seems the nurse came upon these patients in her visitations throughout the neighborhood. How patients interpreted their needs seems to have affected their response to the nurse in these particular cases. Cuts prompted a different reaction than recovery from the rigors of childbirth. In each instance, the exact type of therapeutics provided was determined neither completely from below nor above. Instead, nurses and their patients reached compromises.

Besides revealing the ways in which the nurses scouted for patients, their reports also reveal a larger network of health care providers working in the area. A variety of public and private organizations provided social service assistance in Los Angeles at the turn of the twentieth century. In the absence of a central official authority to coordinate these resources, LACSA took it upon itself to serve as the de facto safety net for the city.

During its existence from 1897 to 1913, LACSA worked regularly with physicians from the city health department, county hospital, medical colleges, and with private practitioners. The College of Medicine—the city's first medical school—became its main associate.[72] Proximity provided one rationale; the college was situated around the corner from LACSA. According to its history, the college chose to locate in the second ward in 1895 because "it [was] in this section of the city that the Mexican and foreign population [was] crowded," providing "an admirable environment to draw from clinical material."[73] Thus, physicians' beliefs about the community appealed to their entrepreneurial and benevolent interests. While LACSA did not characterize their motives for moving to the neighborhood in quite these same terms, they were attracted to the second ward for basically the same reasons. Nearness aside, the settlement also worked with the College of Medicine because in the early 1900s its dispensary served as an important site for the distribution of health care among the poorer residents of Los Angeles.

Formal relationships between the college and the settlement developed at about the same time that Abraham Flexner, an educational reformer, cast skepticism on the value of the college's medical care. (In his now infamous Carnegie-sponsored report on the status of medical education in the United States, Flexner described the clinical laboratory to be "both defective and disorderly" and recommended the school's dissolution.)[74] Despite the college's claimed influence in the neighborhood, its posture was to remain stationary and to wait for patients to seek out its help. LACSA, by contrast, conducted outreach to the community. Although the college established an outpatient obstetrical department in 1903, C. W. Decker noted the expansion of this service once visiting nurses began referring patients and conducting follow-up visits in 1907. Building upon this experience, the college and settlement joined forces to refer patients to the school's general dispensary. According to Decker, LACSA's influence was so important because the settlement sought out the sick in a "systematic" fashion.[75] The story of "H.H." reveals how the nursing association and the college worked together.[76]

One day H.H. missed school because of illness. The school reported his case to LACSA, who sent a nurse to "his home, which [she] found to be two rooms of a rear shack in one of the courts." The nurse found that the boy's ear was "discharging" and because of this he "was frequently out of school." In the minds of settlement workers, a lack of education constituted one of the crucial steps toward a lifetime of delinquency and hence a threat to the stability of society. Hence, this child's ear infection became a public health issue. The nurse "taught [H.H.'s] mother how to keep the ear clean and in a few weeks the ear ceased discharging and he [had] no further trouble with it." The treatment was a success but, more importantly, the nurse believed that in gaining the confidence of H.H.'s mother, her work had greater significance.

During the weeks of her son's treatment, H.H.'s mother began to trust the nurse and eventually revealed "her trouble." Mrs. H.H. "removed the black shawl which she wore over her head and well over her eyes and a pair of smoked glasses" and "exhibited a much inflamed pair of eyes with badly granulated lids." According to the nurse, "they had been sore for so long that they were without eye-winkers and were drawn down at the corners. The head was swollen and cracked in several places and her ears stood stiffly in their swollen condition." Mrs. H.H. did not contest the nurse's desire to send her to the dispensary, where she was diagnosed with eczema. The doctors sent her home with medicine for both her head and eyes, which the nurse helped her administer. The nurse brought science into the home, "impressing upon [Mrs. H.H.] the necessity of thoroughly cleaning the head before using the medicines." Once this was communicated, the nurse noted that she "was very faithful in carrying out the directions." Her head healed first. Upon returning to the dispensary "the doctor who gave her eyes one treatment at the time we began to treat her head, could hardly believe his eyes upon seeing the new growth of hair," exclaiming, "why, that woman was bald when she was here last!" Working together, at least according to their records, LACSA's nurses and the College of Medicine's physicians managed to gain the public's trust.

Besides the College of Medicine, LACSA worked with a number of different private institutions—religiously affiliated and nonsectarian—devoted to issues of social welfare. For instance, in her eleventh report, Weston specifically mentioned that the nurses had worked in conjunction with the Los Angeles City Mission Society (an Episcopalian organization) and the Helping Station of the Anti-Tuberculosis League. Although she did not describe in greater detail LACSA's relationship with the following list of societies, she repeatedly thanked them in her acknowledgments: the Needlework Guild, the Playground Commission, the Assistance League, the Humane Society, the Woman's Auxiliary of St. Matthias Church, and the Junior Auxiliary of St. John's Church.

The most involved relationship LACSA developed with any private organization besides the College of Medicine was with another settlement, the Bethlehem Institute. Founded in 1892 by Reverend Francis M. Price, this Congregational settlement house established a dispensary in 1898 at its "Mother House," 5100 Vignes Street, in the city's eighth ward.[77] According to LACSA, the region contained "the most congested housing and fiercest poverty" in the city.[78]

They also characterized the area as populated by immigrants from Japan, Russia, and "a goodly number of Jews." They were not alone in their depictions of this region as a locale for reform. In detailing the work of Brownson House, a Catholic settlement house located in the area, Mary J. Workman described the eighth ward as such: "Instead of ancient verdure, one sees now the squalid tenements of the poor, one sees the streets full of ragged children of foreign aspect, one sees men and women in the strange garb of foreign peasants continually passing to and fro, and one hears the constant echo of foreign tongues."[79]

In 1908, Reverend Dana Bartlett found the demands of running the dispensary too great for the Bethlehem Institute to handle alone. He held a conference with LACSA and four physicians, two of whom were affiliated with the College of Medicine. They agreed to take over the administration of the dispensary for a test period of six months. Bartlett desired a "systematic service" and, consequently, it was decided to keep the dispensary open five days a week between 1 and 2 P.M. In addition, LACSA appointed one of its nurses to facilitate. Described by Weston as "telling," in the first two months the dispensary reportedly treated 479 patients, roughly 12 per day. Weston believed that these numbers demonstrated a pressing need for health services. The numbers also helped support the continuation of this coordinated effort between the Bethlehem Institute, the local medical community, and LACSA for the next five years.[80]

H.H. and his mother's story began with a recounting of how a school contacted the settlement about an absent pupil. The nurse's report regarding "Mrs. H.," a tubercular victim whose house burned down, also made specific reference to the public schools. According to the nurse, the principal of the Ann Street School "sent clothing for the children" when she learned of the family's plight.[81] These anecdotes were indicative of the amiable and informal relationship LACSA maintained with the public schools. Building on these connections, LACSA began sending the nurse to work in the Amelia and Macy Street schools in 1903. According to LACSA, "Heads are cleaned, contagious skin diseases are carefully investigated, bruises are treated, ears and eyes examined, and instruction in hygiene is given." They also investigated the homes of absentees to determine if "any hidden contagion" was lurking.[82] In these ways, the nurses' proactive assistance differed from that of health officials who came to the schools to inspect the buildings and the students for contagious diseases. Inspection led to suspensions that some parents did not understand while others took offense.[83]

In providing a public health nurse for Los Angeles's public schools, LACSA quickly determined that this work deserved a separate appointment. In 1903, the nurse visited the Amelia and Macy Street schools twenty times, where she attended to 121 children and administered 243 treatments.[84] Subsequently, Weston began bombarding chief health officer Luther Milton Powers with statistics and reports to demonstrate the necessity of school nurses.[85] As a result of her actions and given the resistance he encountered from residents to his staff, Powers appointed LACSA's nurse to attend to six of the city's schools in 1904. She made 132 visits, gave 1,253 treatments, and visited an additional 159 children in their homes. This was in addition to her regular district nursing duties. The work was clearly overwhelming.

By the summer, LACSA requested that the city's board of health shoulder the administrative and fiscal responsibility and appoint nurses whose sole focus would be to work in the public schools. In his health report, Powers suggested that this was his idea.[86] The board looked favorably upon the request, admiring the nurse's ability to help with common afflictions ranging from common colds to the elimination of lice: "These nurses look after the children who are found with sore eyes, running ears, discharging ulcerations, etc., or, in the case of children afflicted with vermin, the nurses go to their homes, and help the mother exterminate the pests. In many cases of minor accidents the nurse can be of great service to the schools."[87] The appeal was successful, and in September the city appointed a nurse to attend to the public schools. According to Yssabella Waters's research, this made Los Angeles the second municipality in the nation to employ a school nurse; New York's board of health appointed a school nurse in 1902.[88] It was also the first step in changing the official structure of the health department in relation to nursing. Unlike the previous arrangement with LACSA, this time the city asked the chief health officer to be the manager.

Despite the new appointment, LACSA decided to keep attending to the three schools closest to the settlement. Powers apparently did not object. Although the nurses reported directly to the settlement, these reports were then "regularly taken to the city health office." By 1911, there were eight school nurses, five under direct supervision of the health department and three from the college settlement. They attended to over 115 schools in the greater Los Angeles area with a total enrollment of 52,054 students.[89]

The health department's willingness to share responsibility for student health with LACSA was one indication of their collaborative abilities. All of the evidence indicates that since the program's inception, LACSA maintained a cordial relationship with the city's health department. Powers had supported their initial petition in 1897 with a handwritten note stating: "I most earnestly recommend that the request of the petitioners be granted."[90] Two years later, Powers lent support when the settlement came under attack from its neighbors. In response, when Weston included an acknowledgment section at the end of her annual reports, she always thanked Powers and the city health department. In contrast, a similar reference to the board of health never appeared. Judging by the minutes of the board of health, the two institutions did not interact with any regularity. Although supportive of LACSA's push for a school nurse, the combined absence of recorded communications and snippets of evidence from 1909 suggest the existence of a greater tension between LACSA and the city's official health policy makers (the board of health) versus its administrators of public health (Powers and the city health department). In 1909, a measles epidemic led all of these entities to rethink the place of public health nursing in Los Angeles.

Without an annual report from the city health department for 1909 and 1910, it is difficult to assess the course and severity of the epidemic. In mid-February of 1910, the board of health stated that there had been over two thousand cases in January and another fifteen hundred since the beginning of the month.[91] Judging by LACSA's account of the event and a report produced by the local media, the initial outbreak appears to have occurred between late October and early November 1909. According to the *Los Angeles Times*, the epidemic was concentrated in the ninth ward in Boyle Heights between the streets of Utah and Anderson.[92] More specifically, the outbreak initially appeared to be limited to a few house courts populated by Russian immigrants. Although they did not provide figures, they claimed that these structures were "packed." (See chapter 2 for a discussion of house courts.) The strain of measles proved particularly virulent, killing twelve out of fourteen patients under the supervision of the health department by the first week of November. Despite afflicting forty children within these few blocks, the health department decided not to invoke its power to quarantine. It left the reason unstated but its comments regarding Russians suggest that the officials believed this group would have protested such a step. In statements reminiscent of Weston's remarks, chief health officer Powers declared that "we have not only a virulent disease . . . but we are dealing with a virulent people."[93] He blamed the health department's inability "to bring a sympathetic relation between the officials and the colonists" on this immigrant group's "natural suspicion of officials." He further suggested that they "seem[ed] perverse to all dictations." Given their widespread publicity, Powers would undoubtedly have been familiar with the riots caused by disagreements over Milwaukee's response to smallpox in immigrant neighborhoods in the 1890s.[94] Attempting to avoid similar turmoil, officials in Los Angeles resolved to acquire nurses to go door-to-door to provide assistance and identify more cases.

In this way, private and public administration joined to meet the crisis. Weston recalled how the association volunteered the services of two nurses to assist with the outbreak and argued that it "was an excellent illustration of 'team work'—physician, nurse, and settlement worker united to fight an epidemic."[95] This contradicts a newspaper account at the time. The *Los Angeles Times* suggested that this relationship was not easily entered into: "It was intimated that the settlement nurses might not submit to the direction of the health authorities."[96] The press did not provide any further indication as to who made the insinuation or why. The fear that LACSA might not cooperate hinted at a larger debate about the quasi-public status of LACSA's program that had begun a few months prior to the measles outbreak. The question before the board of health and the city council was whether the city should incorporate a bureau of nursing into its official city health infrastructure.

In 1912, Weston argued "private appropriations demonstrate needs: but must eventually give way to the legitimate privileges and claims of the Municipality."[97] Through her annual reports, Weston had made a case for the program's necessity. The program's work made health problems visible and highlighted the importance of public health nursing for protecting the public's health in Los Angeles. The council's desire to use LACSA's nurses to cope with the measles epidemic was a case in point. In 1897, Weston argued that LACSA was best suited to supervise the program. Fifteen years later, Weston contended that the city's rapid urbanization was proving too great a burden for the program's current capabilities. "Los Angeles," she said, "is growing. It is spreading along the riverbed more rapidly than on the heights; it is building the shack as well as the bungalow. And the cheap flat and lodging house? This field is practically untouched." She rhetorically asked, "How is it possible for five nurses to cover the field?"[98] Unable to meet these increasing demands, LACSA had turned toward the city in 1909 for a change in status. Questions, however, about its control prevented the immediate creation of an official nursing bureau.

On August 17, 1909, a few months before the measles epidemic occurred, LACSA requested that the board of health consider creating a Commission of Instructive District Nursing. LACSA was probably pleased with the board's initial response. The board voted to send the request to the city's attorney to draw up an ordinance, which the board would then consider at its next regular meeting. It turned out, however, that this issue revealed fissures. Instead of being discussed at the next regular meeting, the ordinance became the subject of a special session two weeks later. Board member Sherwin Gibbons motioned to have the "ordinance providing for a Commission of Instructive District Nursing be rejected." Without a draft of the ordinance, his specific objection is unclear. The good news for the settlement was that Gibbons's motion "was not seconded and lost." Furthermore, the board appointed a subcommittee to speak with the city attorney about creating an ordinance "to comply strictly with the District Nursing as it had been done in the past." No official action on the subject appears to have been taken for another four months. In the meantime, the city experienced the virulent outbreak of measles.

As explained previously, the city turned to LACSA for nurses to attend to those afflicted with measles in the ninth ward. LACSA had already had one nurse working in the area and agreed to appoint a second. In her annual report, Weston argued that this had been a wonderful example of institutional cooperation. Her portrait of events, however, is not in complete accordance with the board of health minutes from the time. Judging by the board's records, the epidemic had not completely subsided when LACSA decided to withdraw its support for the second nurse. If anything, the outbreak was spreading. LACSA sent a message to the board on December 30, stating that Mrs. Silverthorn could no longer act as the city's "special Nurse to look after the unquarantinable contagious diseases."[99] Battling the measles without LACSA's help, the board of health returned to the question of who should have the power over public health nursing in the city. At the next meeting of the board of health on January 18, 1910, it sent a "communication to the City Council asking them to transfer nurses working at present under the Settlement Assc. to the Board of Health."[100] Unlike the previous entries in the minute book, this one did not make reference to an ordinance.

The board's personnel had not changed, but its support for LACSA had. Left unrecorded in the archives is evidence that would illuminate exactly what occurred between the session in August 1909, when the board recommended that the city keep LACSA's program intact, and January 1910, when it appeared to ask for the sole power to govern the nurses. At the end of the month, the board met in the mayor's office for a special session and heard from George H. Kress, a leader of the local medical community.[101] No one from LACSA was present. Kress's objections suggest that the disagreement over the transfer of the program boiled down to whether LACSA or anyone other than a physician would continue to have influence over health policies related to public health nursing.

Kress represented the Los Angeles County Medical Society in opposing lay participation in medical affairs. He argued, "none of the men present at any of its meetings stated his belief that it would be good policy, or proper principle, to let such work be done under the Board of Laymen or of Lay Women." According to Kress, these physicians "were all willing to acknowledge that the College Settlement Association had done a great deal of loyal and effective work in the past and that a certain amount of credit, perhaps, should be given to the College Settlement members for bringing the work up to its present state of completion." Nonetheless, Kress contended that the settlement workers should now concede all authority to physicians in matters of public health. He argued that the "medical men" believed that "in as much as the City is paying the bills we see no reason why your Board should not have the supervision of the work." The gendered subtext of Kress's argument reveals a competition between those who might otherwise be considered interested in the same types of reform. Who had the greater authority in questions of health care, medical men or municipal housekeepers?

Kress might have also had a more personal motivation in opposing LACSA's continued participation in public health policy. He had suffered a personal slight. Kress headed the Tubercular Association and, in 1909, he persuaded the Los Angeles City Council to provide a nurse for his organization. But instead of consigning control over to Kress, the council placed the nurse under the direct supervision of the health department. Kress acknowledged, "As a charitable organization we did not have the right to tell her what to do, although we were willing to co-operate." The settlement's success in solely commanding city funds in contrast to his failure might have fueled his antagonistic attitude.

Kress's plea swayed the board and it unanimously voted to send the following message to the city council: "The Health Board most emphatically protests against the creation of a Commission for the control of district nursing." This still left the board with the problem of what to do about the measles epidemic. They continued to desire public health nurses. On February 15, they composed a message to the city council wherein they argued the detrimental effects on the public's health due to lack of nursing care: "We feel that had we had sufficient nurses the present epidemic of measles could have been in some degree lessened. . . . We also feel that the present way of taking care of indigent contagious cases is inhuman, as aside from the visits of the Health Officers these cases have absolutely no nursing care." The board asked the city council "to create the positions of four additional nurses under the Health Dept."[102]

As a result of these deliberations, LACSA kept its program intact and the city slowly created a place for nursing within its health department. The board of health did not get four nurses but it did get one. In 1910, the department created a position of "special city nurse" and employed a professional nurse, Margaret F. Sirch, to visit maternity hospitals, children's institutions, and boarding homes.[103] She also supervised the school nurse and the tuberculosis nurse. Sirch later called this work "instructive inspection."[104] In these ways, the department's use of nurses did not conflict with LACSA's program. By hiring nurses to focus on specific diseases or tasks, the city's arrangement reflected a growing national trend within public health nursing toward specialization.

Tensions between the board and LACSA over the future of public health nursing appear to have been relieved when the board's influence over these types of decisions came to an abrupt halt in 1911. The city reorganized its charter and abolished the board of health. In its place, the city turned the chief health officer into the city's chief policy maker and administrator, calling the new position "health commissioner." This was good news for the settlement because since 1897, LACSA had found an ally in Powers. It is reasonable to conclude that his consistent support helps explain why there is an absence of recorded objection to an ordinance establishing a Bureau of District Nursing within the Health Department in 1913 that allowed female reformers to maintain an official role in crafting public health policy.

By a unanimous vote and without debate, the city council adopted ordinance No. 27,742 on June 10, 1913. It established a Bureau of Municipal Nursing within the health department of the city of Los Angeles. In turning the program over to the city, the settlement expressed its sentiments in a letter, which representatives read to the mayor and council of the city of Los Angeles prior to the presentation and adoption of the ordinance. The settlement stated that this action "fulfill[ed] a long-cherished plan." These women did not see this transfer as a break. Instead, from their point of view, they had always viewed public health nursing as a civic responsibility. Their letter recounted how the nursing program combined both the art of sympathy with scientific ideals, and expressed hope that the program's integrity would be maintained by the amalgamation.[105]

The settlement did more than hope. The ordinance provided a structural means through which female reformers could preserve their influence. By this law, a nursing commission would run the new bureau. The commission was to be composed of five people, of which no more than three could be of one sex and no more than three could be physicians or nurses. Thus, "lay" and "medical" control would be counterbalanced and presumably allow the women of LACSA to maintain some measure of power over policy. Appointed by the health commissioner, the commissioners could not serve more than four years consecutively (although this rule appears to have been ignored). The committee members also worked without compensation. The commission remained in place until the city instituted a new charter in 1924. In the reorganization of the city's public health infrastructure, a board of health was reestablished and the ordinance forming the bureau was allowed to expire.

Although the structure of the commission would have allowed LACSA to maintain a presence in directing public health policy related to nursing, it appears that its members did not actually play a direct role. Instead, female commissioners were most often clubwomen.[106] Despite the absence of settlement workers, in these other ways women still retained an important influence. In fact, this type of arrangement was common practice in other visiting nurse organizations.

The newly created Bureau of Municipal Nursing combined the settlement's nursing association with the health department's disparate nursing programs that it had begun to develop when it appointed a school nurse in 1903. Since that time, the city had added to its staff a nurse to work with indigent tubercular patients and a "special" nurse whose job it was to conduct inspections of institutions related to child welfare. The bureau provided for the inspection of public and parochial schools, inspection of children's homes and institutions, and inspection of hospitals and midwives, all previously duties of the special nurse. It also created a division for district nursing, maternity nursing, and infant welfare stations, all previously part of LACSA's program. Weston did not accompany her organization. Instead, she consigned control over to the city's special nurse, Margaret F. Sirch, thus allowing a professional nurse to take charge of management. The bureau continued to offer job opportunities for public health nurses in Los Angeles, it continued to offer health care services to the city's poorer classes, and it continued to blur public and private because the commission directed public health policy.

In coping with demographic changes in the 1920s, officials responded by modifying the program's organization. When the nursing bureau was incorporated in 1913, it was divided into a number of specialties including the inspection of schools, children's homes, hospitals, maternity cases, tuberculosis cases, and infant welfare stations. According to the chief of the bureau, Margaret F. Sirch, the rapid growth of the city created inefficiency and situations of endangerment.[107] Sometimes the nurses entirely missed potential cases. Sirch advocated replacing this division of labor with a more generalized service based on region rather than specific assignments. She argued that "the community nurse has a distinct advantage in knowing her families and only in proportion as a nurse becomes familiar with her locality does her value increase." In addition, Sirch urged that the "saving of time and car fare demand[ed]" consolidation. Sirch claimed that this type of reorganization had already "worked out very satisfactorily in several eastern cities and is considered by experts to be by far the most efficient plan for public health nursing." Sirch's plan was laid aside when she resigned to take a position in the California State Board of Charities and Corrections. Two years later, however, the city adopted a similar proposal.

Having commissioners made a difference in shaping the future of public health nursing in Los Angeles. While other cities allowed health officials who were unschooled in the principles and practicalities of public health nursing to dictate policy, the commission brought in a national leader of the profession, Mary E. Lent, to restructure the city's nursing bureau in 1916. Lent had established the Instructive Visiting Nurse Association of Baltimore in 1906, and had just been appointed associate secretary of the National Organization for Public Health Nursing. She worked for six months constructing a plan, which was then adopted by the city. Her strategy was to eliminate distinctions among tuberculosis, district, and school nursing. She promoted the use of a public health nurse to attend to families as a unit.[108] Contemporaries described Lent's Los Angeles plan as having "never been surpassed."[109] Even after the city rewrote its charter in 1924 and changed the structure of its public health administration, Lent's plan for public health nursing remained intact. In sticking with Lent's design to keep a program of practical nursing as well as educational services, Los Angeles did not follow the path of other health departments in eschewing home care.[110] In continuing both aspects, Los Angeles preserved a program that bore a closer resemblance to its predecessor than that of other cities.

Whereas discarded in other cities, public health nursing remains an integral part of the city's health system to this day. The program still provides routine care to the city's most vulnerable residents. Its origins stem from the activities of female reformers at the end of the nineteenth century. Working outside of the city's official bureaucratic structure, they devised ways to shape the course of health care delivered in the city by pressuring officials to revise their stance on providing medical services for its residents in their homes. Residents in Los Angeles made use of these services and in their acceptance or resistance affected LACSA's program. The establishment of LACSA's public health nursing program proved to be the first in a series of formal engagements by female reformers in constructing and influencing the distribution of civic health services.

Chapter 2

Public Authority for a Private Program
Housing Reform

Developing a public health nursing program put the Los Angeles College Settlement Association (LACSA) in people's homes. From these experiences, settlement workers became aware of housing conditions that they considered hazardous to health. Yet, until Jacob Riis visited the city in January 1905 and allegedly said that Los Angeles had "congested slums, as bad, . . . if not as extensive, as anything to be found in New York City," LACSA did not organize a movement defined solely for housing reform.[1] In the beginning, LACSA's work in public health nursing provided qualitative and quantitative information about housing conditions. Later, the public nurse came to serve as a model for the ideal housing inspector. Yet, in contrast to its public health nursing program, LACSA developed a much stronger cooperative relationship with other reform organizations to promote housing reform and gradually receded from a leadership role to a supporting one. Unlike public health nursing, reformers did not conceive of housing as a particularly feminine subject of concern. Nonetheless, women's organizations, especially women's clubs and settlement workers, played a pivotal part in expanding municipal public health services.

Turn-of-the-twentieth century reformers viewed "the housing problem" as both a physical and a moral issue.[2] Their concerns about the structure of living space intertwined with issues of work and leisure. They came to label certain types of dwellings—lodging houses and hotels that housed working-class individuals—as deviant in their essence rather than form. They came to focus on tenements as the only redeemable spaces to expend their energies and eventually government money. Reformers explicitly interested in housing focused on domiciles they believed would perpetuate the institution of the nuclear family in the face of modernity. As Jacob Riis stated in 1891, "The family home is the basis upon which our modern civilization rests."³ Single men and women sat outside their construction of family or were viewed as being in a transitory state from which they would eventually come to rest in a nuclear family structure. This assumption about domestic architecture had not always existed.⁴ Still, by the turn of the twentieth century this division influenced housing reform in Los Angeles. Despite public health officials continued interest in lodging houses and hotels, city efforts initially focused on "house courts"—single-storied row houses of one to three rooms that shared communal sewage and water facilities and were typically of cheap wooden construction—because to the members of LACSA the presence of married women and their children flagged these structures as sites for transformation.

Household relationships constituted only one indicator to reformers. Geographical space became imbued with ethnic meaning during this period: slums became not just spaces of the poor but spaces of the immigrant poor. Historical discussions of turn-of-the-twentieth-century housing highlight the relationship between ethnicity, racism, and housing structures.⁵ Prior to the 1920s, reformers in Los Angeles turned their attention to house courts partly because of the polyglot of immigrant groups who lived within them.

LACSA's leaders, however, did not define hazardous living conditions only by the ethnicity of the tenants. Instead, they spoke the language of late-nineteenth-century public health sanitarians who believed that a lack of light, air, and access to clean facilities generated unhealthy living conditions no matter who lived inside. At various times these women also made use of the new scientific language of germs to promote housing reform, but they did this in confluence with arguments about sanitation. This is not surprising in light of Nancy Tomes's research on the "private side of public health," which demonstrates the ways in which middle-class women embraced their new roles as household health guardians battling simultaneously against dirt and germs.⁶

That Riis surprised the public with his statement became an important part of the legend of housing reform in Los Angeles. Yet, in retrospect, housing reformers noted several factors that made it very unsurprising that the city possessed slums. The expansion of the railroads, manufacturing interests, and a general real estate boom fueled economic opportunities that attracted tens of thousands of migrants. According to the U.S. Census, the population of Los Angeles doubled from 1890 to 1900 and tripled from 1900 to 1910 (50,395 to 102,479 to 319,198). In a mere thirty years, Los Angeles jumped from the fifty-seventh to the seventeenth most populous city in the United States.⁷

Scholars have long commented on the dominance of middle-class native-born Midwesterners' migration to the city and their occupation of bungalows as a crucial aspect setting Los Angeles's urbanization apart from other cities during the turn of the twentieth century.[8] Yet the city also attracted working-class migrants from southern and eastern Europe, numerically the major groups migrating to the United States in the Progressive Era. In sheer numbers, the foreign-born population in Los Angeles increased fivefold between 1890 and 1910, rising from 12,753 to 60,584.

In discussing issues of housing in the East and Midwest, urban reformers described an influx of foreign-born immigrants into particular neighborhoods. U.S. Census figures for Los Angeles from 1890 and 1900 allow some comparison because they detail population growth by wards. At first glance, it appears that Los Angeles did not experience what its metropolitan counterparts did. Instead of clustering in particular neighborhoods, the U.S. Census figures indicate that Los Angeles's foreign-born population was more evenly spread out in 1900 than it was in 1890. Still, the wards that attracted reformers' attentions (2, 7, 8, and 9) continued to house large numbers of the foreign born.[9] The downtown area was a diverse ethnic mixture during this period.[10] Hence, whether or not Los Angeles experienced the same growth strains as its metropolitan counterparts, the perception of reformers was that the city had "some excuse for slum districts" and associated those areas with working-class immigrants.[11]

Local clubwomen and settlement workers became engaged in issues of environmental reform related to housing prior to Jacob Riis's visit to Los Angeles in January 1905. In fact, Riis's negative comment about Los Angeles was not even the first of this sort. As discussed in the introduction, James Bronson Reynolds, the chief executive of the New York University Settlement, had stood before the women of the Friday Morning Club (FMC) in 1894 and pronounced Los Angeles to be in an abysmal state. Nor was Riis's lecture the first possible formal exposure FMC members might have had to discussions about the built environment. In March of 1895, Miss M. M. Fette presented a lecture to the FMC on "Municipal Housekeeping," wherein she discussed "The Tenement House, Saloon, Pawn Shop, and Other Plague Spots in our Cities."[12] Although she did not talk about Los Angeles—she compared "the object lessons of the reform work of London, Birmingham, Glasgow, and Berlin"—her talk still related to local conditions because she linked social reform to political change. (Fette's talk coincided with the emergence of a new movement for suffrage in California, a movement that utilized the idea of "civic activism" to argue for formal political inclusion.)[13] According to the club's records, Fette "illustrate[d] the influence of women [in altering urban settings], when granted municipal suffrage on equal footing with [men]." Just a few months later, women in Los Angeles interested in reform engaged in civic activism with respect to the environment. In May 1895, members of LACSA conducted a survey of the sanitary conditions of one of the oldest areas of the city—Sonoratown—after which they relayed their findings to the city's board of health and successfully argued for the appointment of a female health inspector to address their concerns.

Beyond these brief clues into what female reformers might have heard or did in the mid-1890s about environmental conditions related to housing, their descriptions of early settlement activities make it clear that female reformers in Los Angeles were cognizant of a relationship between urban environments and health. Three years after establishing LACSA in 1894, the institution published its first report documenting its history and activities. The opening vignette took readers on a virtual tour of Sonoratown, which conjured associations between geography, immigrants, and disease. LACSA began by recounting the story of Marie Geantit, whose residence became the future site of the settlement. Geantit—a widowed Frenchwoman who had settled in southern California in the 1850s, where she appears to have acted as a petty merchant—moved to Sonoratown because she "had always hoped that Sonoratown would be the most attractive part of the city."[14] According to LACSA, Geantit had taken measures to make this a reality. For instance, she had "laid before her doors the first stone sidewalk which had ever been seen in Los Angeles." LACSA used the story of Geantit's residential experience to argue that the growth of the modern city fostered feelings of disassociation: "But the city had passed her by, stretching itself for miles on either side of her toward mountain and sea, with its thousands of people and hurrying, restless life. Even her old friends had deserted her, foreigners and indifferent strangers were now her neighbors." A key symbol of this change was the restructuring of Geantit's adobe into a tenement.

What did the women of LACSA consider a "Sonoratown tenement"? It did not have to be several stories high, nor made of brick. Instead, the essential ingredients were a lack of ventilation, absence of light, and, in their opinion, the presence of too many inhabitants. Above all, the structure needed to convey a sense of deterioration. In these respects, their descriptions do not appear all that different from those found in the periodical literature at the time describing other locales.

If members of LACSA read nationally syndicated journals in the 1890s prior to the publication of their report, they would have been aware of an emerging movement to reform housing. Between 1890 and 1897, the *Reader's Guide to Periodical Literature* listed a total of twenty-nine articles related to housing; eight of these related specifically to New York City. The guide also indexed another thirteen articles related to tenements. William T. Elsing, a self-proclaimed "city missionary," asked the central question on reformers' minds: could a home exist in a tenement house?[15] Investigations into conditions rendered similar judgments; tenements were unsafe because they invariably lacked adequate daylight, aeration, and access to facilities. Air-shafts, hallway sinks, and unisex bathrooms all came under attack. Another essential complaint was overcrowding. In some cases reformers demarcated structures as the issue, in others the tenants. The majority emphasized the man-made nature of housing ills and proposed man-made solutions.

In describing the tenements of Sonoratown, LACSA began with exteriors. Nothing about the outside façade of the building, according to LACSA, provided an obvious alarm to viewers that it was a bad house: "You must picture to yourself what the Mexicans call an ideal home. Around three sides of a patio or courtyard a one-storied house was built. It had a few windows and many doors, and the walls, two feet thick, were made of adobe, and were white-washed without and in. But the best part of this home was the patio." It was in these courtyards, LACSA claimed, that señors and señoritas of a prior generation had spent leisurely afternoons napping to soft guitar music with the smell of orange blossoms and roses wafting in the air. Standing in the "miserable" courtyard in 1897, LACSA told viewers that if they looked hard enough they could "see a vestige of past beauty." While "decrepit," an orange tree trunk stood in one corner, and while "dejected," a rose bush stood in another. LACSA used these rhetorical contrasts to impart a historical sense of place and to provide justification for their current endeavors. Relegating adobe into relics to be replaced by brick structures was both a physical and metaphorical process of turning Los Angeles into a modern American city.[16] In order to help readers understand what made this housing stock a site for remediation, LACSA took them inside.

Moving from the exterior to the interior of the adobe, LACSA called attention to its restructuring. The report noted, "The large rooms have been partitioned off into very small ones."[17] Geantit's residence, a single adobe, had "been converted into eleven tenement units." Making a connection between exterior and interior, LACSA argued that the city's infrastructure could not handle the new demands generated by the numbers of individuals living within these structures. LACSA challenged readers to reimagine their perception of Los Angeles from a locale of health resorts to one of health hazards: "Do you feel quite so sure of the health condition of Los Angeles as you did before you saw these courtyards? Do you think malaria and fever may not find breeding places where drains are reeking with refuse, sewage has no outlet and garbage is irregularly gathered?" These comments indicate a familiarity with the science of sanitation in combating disease.

If this was not enough to convince the reader of the settlement's necessity in Sonoratown, LACSA also included descriptions of vice. They noted that saloons existed on "almost every street corner" and that "houses of ill-repute" were nestled among "respectable homes." These settlement workers considered the organization of cityscapes a physical and moral health issue. Although LACSA did not make any explicit rhetorical associations between immigrants and disease, in the same sections of the report where it described the deterioration of structures it saw fit to mention that Mexicans, Italians, French, Bavarians, Germans, Danes, Scotch, Irish, Arabs, and Chinese lived within the area. In sum, in its first published report LACSA combined descriptions of housing conditions, residents, and businesses to justify the necessity of its reform efforts in this specific environment. Housing was not a distinctive issue but part of a larger understanding of environmental reform.

Archival evidence does not yield any direct communications between LACSA and the health department or board of health regarding housing reform before Riis's visit in 1905. Still, the health department's institutional records indicate that it shared some of LACSA's concerns while also having some of its own. The 1890 annual report indicates that health officials had an intimate acquaintance with problems of the urban infrastructure that correlated to housing.[18] For instance, the majority of the city's sewers existed in areas dominated by tenements. Chief health officer Granville MacGowan believed this presented a danger because he felt that landlords failed to provide "ventilation" for the sewers, "so as to prevent the escape of gases into the streets through man holes and into our houses through the traps upon the house drains." MacGowan's report included a map of the sewers that visually indicated the interconnectedness of this public health threat.

LACSA identified malaria and "fever" as two diseases associated with bad housing. Similarly, MacGowan also drew connections between sanitary conditions and diphtheria and typhoid fever. He linked their prevalence to the health department's ability to police sanitary conditions. MacGowan argued that the "reduction of the force of our inspectors, and the consequent inability of the department to make house-to-house inspections in the search for non-sanitary conditions," had led to an increase in diptheria. He was especially upset because he had made significant headway in decreasing the rates of both diseases just the year before, reducing fatalities in diphtheria from sixty to twenty-seven and typhoid fever from thirty-seven to one.

In addition to disease within homes, MacGowan was concerned about the structures themselves. He remarked on the demolition of "many filthy shanties and the erection of handsome brick blocks in their places." The houses in question were "the old tumbledown rookeries of the South side of the plaza" inhabited by Chinese immigrants. According to his report, the health department conducted weekly inspections of Chinatown in order to "keep the Chinese population constantly under surveillance." As Natalia Molina has noted, no white ethnic populations were singled out for such attention during the 1890s.[19] In this case, the health department did not make a distinction between the structures and the occupants as to who or what constituted a hazard to the public's health. Instead, place, people, and disease were interchangeable.

Yet fears of contagion were not limited to Chinatown. Every ward came under scrutiny. The health department inspected sewers, businesses, water services, health care providers, the soil, housing stock, and residents to reach conclusions about risk. In the second ward—the location of Sonoratown—the department noted the existence of "many adobe houses. Mexicans, Italian tenement houses, Chinese. Business blocks and a few hotels." Similarly, the health department described the seventh ward as "thickly settled. Small dwellings, factories, retail business blocks. Many poor Mexicans and Negroes. Many tenement houses greatly crowded." In contrast, the health department omitted mentions of ethnicity and race in its descriptions of the fourth and fifth wards. MacGowan described the fourth ward's housing stock as "residence property for principally richer classes, some business property" and the fifth ward as "residence property for richer classes, mostly isolated dwellings." At first glance, the omission is suggestive of a dichotomy of white and wealth versus people of color and poverty. Yet, before we collapse ethnicity, race, and class together, the health department's descriptions of the third and eighth wards need to be taken into consideration. In neither case did the department indicate population as it did for the second and seventh wards. The department, however, did demarcate class. It described the eastern half of the third ward as containing "residences, hotels, and many boarding houses" and the eighth ward as an area with "many tenement houses greatly crowded."[20] What is instructive about these descriptions is that although health officials found it necessary to indicate where Italians, Chinese, Mexicans, and African Americans lived, their writings suggest that class might have been the most informative category for shaping their perceptions of public health threats during this period. Class directly overlapped with housing stock and disease production in the writings of health officials in 1890 in ways that did not appear in LACSA's descriptions in 1897. Yet, in the end, these two visions converged as housing became understood as a distinct issue for reform.

Since 1908, public health officials and historians have paraphrased and publicized Riis's comment that Los Angeles had "congested slums, as bad, . . . if not as extensive, as anything to be found in New York City."[21] Although archival sources do not offer any direct substantiation that he uttered these words, it is not likely that reformers imagined it. James B. Lane has concluded that Riis frequently enjoyed making these types of pronouncements in cities that portrayed New York as their antithesis.[22] Whether Riis actually issued the comment or not, reformers in the 1900s claimed that his presence played a pivotal role in how they came to understand housing as a distinct public health issue in Los Angeles.

Although LACSA members left no archival evidence of their personal engagement with Jacob Riis during his visit to the city in January 1905, it was in his wake that they reconceived the place of housing within their larger program for reform. In describing their work in Woods's *Handbook* in 1911, LACSA claimed that it instigated housing reform in the city. It contended that "the settlement first brought to notice certain deplorable housing conditions and through its influence and that of the Municipal League a housing commission was created upon which one of its members has served continuously."[23] Similarly, a *Los Angeles Times* article from December 1906 stated that "the housing commission was also the outcome of settlement agitation, the workers taking prominent people from other cities to visit the dreadful courts in their neighborhood and to get advice from those accustomed to grappling with such problems."[24] While LACSA took claim for this civic activism, its members were not the ones who thought to bring Riis to the city. Instead, another women's group was responsible for that action.

Jacob Riis visited Los Angeles at the behest of the Young Women's Christian Association, which seized the opportunity to bring the famous reformer to the city while he was engaged in an extensive lecture tour of the western United States. Fifteen years earlier, his photographic lectures of New York's slums and the publication of *How the Other Half Lives* had formed public health agendas as well as made him a celebrity. Riis publicized to the middle and upper classes of New York the deplorable conditions of the poor and the working class in their midst. He documented piles of garbage, the absence of adequate sewage facilities, and the proliferation of contagious disease. Riis believed that these conditions would only get worse unless private citizens sponsored and shaped government intervention. He presented similar arguments in lecturing Los Angelenos, and much of the reform that was to follow in the city used his model of advocacy.

Riis appears to have arrived in Los Angeles on Tuesday, January 3, 1905. He presented his lecture "Slum Life in the Great Cities" to a packed audience of over thousand at the Simpson Auditorium. Reporters were unimpressed by

Riis's stature. The *Los Angeles Times* remarked on his foreign accent, and the *Los Angeles Examiner* on his lack of eloquence.[25] Yet the newspapers also offered insights into the man's mystique: "His manifest soul absorption in his work on the redemption of humanity held the audience for nearly two hours." The *Times* highlighted this point by printing a drawing of Riis gesturing, as if making an emphatic point, to accompany the article. Riis's dedication, as well as his pictures and descriptions of New York's slums, captured the attention of Los Angeles.

According to the *Los Angeles Times*, "the audience shuddered when the speaker showed a block of tenement houses [in New York] that contained the homes of 5,000 persons and said there was not a bathtub in the place. Then, it burst into a laugh when he corrected himself and admitted he had made a misstatement." What followed next must have hushed the audience. One bathtub did exist. Furthermore, this one tin tub did not fit into anybody's home, instead it hung in an airshaft only twenty-seven inches wide. Riis argued that New York's authorities had exhibited an early complacency toward slum conditions and had only responded when epidemics of cholera created crisis situations. Characterizing New York's tenements as "infant slaughter-houses" and suggesting that "the animal fits better into the landscape" than people, Riis vividly portrayed the importance and possibilities for public health reform.

The public in Los Angeles responded to Riis's testimony by arranging for a second lecture later in the week. Although the second talk, entitled "Tony's Hardships," presumably continued the same graphic themes as the first, the *Los Angeles Herald* claimed that it would appeal "not only to the mother and fathers but to the children as well."[26] Whether it became a family affair is unclear. What is apparent, however, is that Riis's second talk met with as much success as the first, bringing "forth rounds of applause from the enthusiastic audience."[27]

Jacob Riis impressed Los Angelenos, but was it mutual? His tour included stops in Pasadena, Redlands, Riverside, and Ventura, and the local press reported that he found the area "better than paradise."[28] Although Riis did not specifically mention Los Angeles in his letters to family and friends, his personal papers corroborate the newspapers' accounts regarding his general impression of southern California.[29] Spending time first in northern California, which he found wet and cold, Riis hoped to find sunshine in the south. Apparently Mother Nature acquiesced. Writing to friend Lyman Powell, Riis declared "what anybody wants to *live out* of Southern California for I don't understand. Most assuredly when I am dead I will live there often, if my astral body takes to sunshine." In addition, Riis partook in the purported benefits of the southern California climate by retiring to a sanitarium in Santa Barbara for the latter half of January after his visit to Los Angeles.[30]

Although it appears that Riis's rhetorical effervescence was genuine, it also served a practical purpose. Besides being a means to raise social consciousness, his lecture series was also a fund-raising expedition. Speaking to the *Los Angeles Times*, Riis said, "What I hope will come to pass . . . is that we can find capitalists who will be willing to invest $100,000 if necessary in rebuilding the tenements of New York and to be satisfied with an income of 3 or 4 percent on the investment."[31] Unlike his characterizations of southern California, his plea for money might not have been so appealing. It was less than half of what investors could make in the local real-estate market.[32]

Riis's personal accounting records do not indicate whether he succeeded in finding investors, but he did fulfill his other objective. Contemporaries later characterized his visit as an "awakening" that "jarred the complacency" of Los Angeles.[33] Despite positive publicity at the time, local reformers would later recount a different story about Riis's impressions of their city. Yet it took more than a visit from Riis to turn interest into a movement. At least two other events played a role in prompting action. In the winter, the Women's Civic Federation (WCF) set out to change garbage collection, and, in the summer, another famous reformer, Graham Taylor, paid the city a visit.[34] More than discuss the relationship between environment and disease, the WCF and Taylor directly challenged citizens about their own inactivity.

In late February 1905, a month and a half after Riis's visit, the WCF agitated to transform the way the city collected its garbage (the contract was due to expire August 1).[35] As "householders in the city of Los Angeles," it objected to the sight of "half-spilled garbage can[s], festering on the sidewalk in the public view at all hours of the day." The WCF attributed the problem to the city's growth. It argued that urbanization had transformed the city's housing stock, especially in the number of multifamily dwellings. The increase in apartment houses, according to the WCF, led to "unsightly decorations of the sidewalks on the day set aside for the collection of garbage. The display . . . is a sight for the gods." It petitioned the city to arrange for garbage to be picked up at night and argued that the spectacle of garbage on the streets during the day was not only "disgusting" but "a disgrace to us in the opinion of visitors from all parts of the world." Garbage, the women argued, made an unfavorable impression on tourists. As "householders," if not as property owners, these women asserted that they had a stake in the city's status.

The WCF sent the petition to other women's clubs, asking them to sign in support. This request met with success. The Friday Morning Club, Ebell, and

Wednesday Morning Club signed, as did the Ruskin Art Club and Landmarks Club. In addition, chief health commissioner L. M. Powers, the Municipal League, and the Merchants and Manufacturers' Association also promised to back the WCF.

Although part of the WCF's claim was that the garbage situation was an aesthetic offense, the organization moved beyond aestheticism to argue that the situation was a matter of public safety. In its petition to the city, the WCF contended, "garbage exposed to the almost perpetual sun of our climate unquestionably breeds disease." It claimed that "here, heated by the burning sun [the garbage cans] emit fumes that are not only offensive, but which actually smote the little children passing to and from school, with the germs of disease." The *Los Angeles Times* helped to emphasize this aspect by accompanying the article with drawings of vapors rising from garbage cans. Using overlapping rhetoric of miasmas and germs, the WCF underscored the point that disease and garbage were interrelated. It also argued that Los Angeles's distinct climate created distinct risks.

The WCF was only one source of inspiration. Graham Taylor, a leader in the social settlement movement in Chicago, visited in the summer. After he left, the *Los Angeles Times* reported that during his trip he had "inspect[ed] . . . the Los Angeles congested district, and . . . declar[ed] that, while limited in its area, in many ways it is as bad as the conditions which prevail in Chicago."[36] Although this comment presumably packed as much punch as Riis's, housing reformers did not refer to Taylor's statement in detailing their history. Unlike the evidence available for Riis, however, it is clear that Taylor had direct contact with leaders from LACSA and the Municipal League, the two groups that officially took up housing reform with city bureaucrats.

Taylor left his Chicago home in the summer of 1905 to visit the Pacific Coast. He toured both cities and nature. His route took him through Yosemite, Portland, Berkeley, Oakland, San Jose, Los Angeles, and the Grand Canyon before returning to Chicago.[37] Those who read the *Los Angeles Times* religious section would have known of his impending arrival in southern California and learned about his social settlement, the Chicago Commons.[38] Taylor spent four days in Los Angeles in the middle of August. Judging from his diary of daily activities, he spent more time with Dana Bartlett of the Bethlehem Institute, a Congregational settlement in the eighth ward, than with other reformers in Los Angeles. Still, Taylor recorded dining with one of the Stoddarts at Casa de Castelar (LACSA's original name) and lunching with Charles Dwight Willard from the Municipal League.[39] On his last day, LACSA joined together with the Brownson House and Bethlehem Institute to provide Taylor with a final reception.[40]

Taylor delivered numerous speeches during his visit. In addition to speaking twice at the Bethlehem Institute, Taylor spoke at the First Congregational Church, the First Methodist Church, the Minister's Union, and the Masonic Hall.[41] According to the *Los Angeles Times*, although the Social Gospel—a movement to use Christian tenets to achieve salvation for society instead of focusing on personal redemption—remained the mainstay of his message, Taylor adjusted his talks to his audiences. The *Times* reported that his talk to the First Congregational Church, entitled "The Social Incarnation," differed in tone from the one given to the "neighboring people" assembled in the "parlors of the men's hotel" at the Bethlehem Institute who gathered to listen to Taylor speak on the subject of "Democracy and Religion." The *Times* claimed that Taylor changed his public persona from a "dignified minister who spoke formally from the pulpit" to a "businessman addressing his associates and planning the best methods of procedure." Although the newspaper did not report on the activities that occurred the following evening at the Masonic Hall, they believed that his talk to "labor-union people" would prompt an "animated" discussion.

Although Taylor's log of activities do not provide any more specifics on his impressions of the "congested district," at least one contemporary newspaper article indicates that he was paying attention to Los Angeles's housing situation. According to the *Los Angeles Times*, Taylor singled out Bartlett's work in providing housing for transient men as exceptional: "I have never seen before a men's hotel or lodging-house with the home atmosphere." He believed Bartlett's work should be supported, extended, and serve as a model for other cities. Yet Taylor also still believed that even the best lodging house was "done at great cost to family life."[42] The primacy of reformers' concern to establish dwellings within which "family life" would be promoted encouraged them to set aside any great agitation for alternative forms of housing.[43]

It is unclear exactly when LACSA decided to pursue a typical Progressive Era reform strategy and ask the mayor to appoint a special commission to investigate housing conditions in the city.[44] What the settlement did not do, which was common elsewhere, was to conduct an initial door-to-door query to document conditions. An extensive investigation was unnecessary because LASCA's public health nurse already provided data on the areas in question. Thus, instead of generating qualitative and quantitative data to present to the mayor, LACSA jumped straight to publicity.

In attempting to secure favor with the mayor, female reformers worked with the local and national presses to publicize housing as a specific public health hazard in Los Angeles. In late September 1905, a reporter for the

Los Angeles Times ventured out into the "congested districts of the Second, Eighth, and Ninth wards of Los Angeles" and argued that his "investigation" turned up "some startling conditions constantly menacing the sanitary welfare of the city."[45] Although the reporter portrayed him or herself as acting alone (no authorship is given), by the reporter's remarks it seems likely that he or she contacted LACSA during the investigation and perhaps toured the area with its nurse.

The reporter attempted to sway readers and municipal officials to take civic action through a variety of inflammatory arguments and visuals. For instance, the reporter referenced eugenics when elaborating on the conditions in the "congested districts," declaring that "no race suicide" exists in the eighth ward, where "Mexican, Russians, and Italians" all appeared to this reporter to reproduce prodigiously. Six photographs accompanied the article and the captions left little to the reader's imagination: "houses of diphtheria germs," "just arrived," "all nations," "twelve families and butcher shop in this building," and "living in horse stalls." While it was clear from Graham Taylor's visit and the WCF's comments that a variety of housing structures were at issue, the *Times* reporter focused on house courts, specifically "Castelar Court." (This also appears to be the first time the term "house court" appears in print.) The reporter described it as being only two lots wide, composed of thirty dwellings—the majority were one-room, some of which had been converted from stables—and inhabited by almost hundred men, women, and children. Rather than blame landlords for inadequate facilities, the reporter felt that the problem stemmed from the "great influx of foreigners" who, he claimed, were "unused to California methods of sanitation, and to the California idea of each family having ample elbow room, with a garden or grass plot, and free access of sunlight and pure air into the living rooms." The reporter warned the public that the rest of the city must constantly "preach [to the immigrants] the gospel of fresh air and cleanliness or the day will surely come when this city will suffer sorely for its sins against the stranger within our gates." In the mind of this reporter, issues of housing, immigration, and modernity converged.

The *Los Angeles Times* reporter claimed that while the health department made "constant attempts" to secure sanitary conditions in these wards, the residents committed "daily violations of the dictates of common sense." The reporter noted how volunteer organizations had come to the health department's aid. The *Times* reporter listed the different groups engaged in ameliorating conditions within these wards: the Bethlehem Institute, the Brownson House, El Hogar Felis, the King's Daughters, and LACSA. Although declining to give specific details about each of these organizations, because the "efforts of each of these institutions would be a story of itself," the reporter made an exception for LACSA's public health nurse. He described her as a "faithful minister to the physical needs of the people" and argued that any who made "the rounds" with her through the community would be spurred into action.

Two months later, in early December 1905, Bessie Stoddart, the secretary of the playground commission and a founding member of LACSA, published the "Courts of Sonoratown," subtitled "The Housing Problem as It Is to Be Found in Los Angeles," in the *Charities and Commons*.[46] This took what was a local issue and gave it national publicity. Unlike the reporter for the *Los Angeles Times*, Stoddart emphasized the need for new laws regarding building structures. She argued that while "the city health officer can inspect and order landlords to clean the courts, but beyond that he has little authority." Similar to the *Times*, she noted the role of LACSA's nurse as an instrument of information for the city. In one case, according to Stoddart, the nurse found "twenty-three sleepers in two tiny rooms." The nurse, she argued, had acted as "a potent agency for the prevention of disease." But Stoddart did not view the nurse as the ultimate solution for ameliorating housing problems. She argued that the city needed to take action. She warned that if it did not "prevent the one-story crowding, and the many-storied crowding which will undoubtedly follow in its wake, we shall indeed be confronted by such conditions as have done incalculable harm in the older cities, and which with just a little foresight and common sense might be prevented here."

Stoddart discussed the science of sanitation and germs to make her case for government action. Similar to the *Los Angeles Times*, she argued that because the tenants had migrated from rural areas they were not familiar with the rules of urban sanitation. In contrast to the reporter, however, Stoddart blamed the landlords for creating structures without floors and adequate facilities that would have offset the immigrants' lack of knowledge of modern plumbing. According to Stoddart, landlord negligence proved deadly. She used the issue of women's health to express her outrage: "When the heavy rains come in winter, imagine those shacks and tents that have no floors! Sick women lie on damp mattresses which are embedded in mud." Stoddart also suggested that problems existed beyond negligent landlords; nature generated its own threats. In this way, the issue of climate was central to her understanding of public health in Los Angeles. In her example, Stoddart made reference to the winter deluges that, while intermittent, occurred every year with certainty. Safe sanitation in the face of winter storms was imperative. Stoddart also used the rhetoric of microbes. She argued, "If it were not for the friendly Southern sun destroying disease germs the day long, frequent epidemics would draw attention to these places of incubation, and better sanitation and housing laws would be enacted." (Her opinion contrasted with that expressed by the WCF, demonstrating the variance in the public's knowledge of the germ theory.) Presumably these powerful images and rhetoric played a role in the mayor's receptivity to appointing a commission.

In retrospect, the Municipal League and LACSA both claimed responsibility for instigating housing reform in Los Angeles, but since no article comparable to Stoddart's appears in the Municipal League's journal or in any documents in Willard's personal papers about the proposed housing commission, it seems reasonable to conclude that LACSA took the lead. In addition, LACSA had been writing about the hazards of housing since 1897. In contrast, the Municipal League's first public stance on the subject occurred in February 1906. It also seems reasonable to believe that LACSA turned to the Municipal League for help. Charles Dwight Willard had founded the Municipal League in 1901 as an organization for persons interested in civic improvement. By 1905, the league consisted of approximately six hundred members and participated in issues of city planning, zoning, and municipal ownership.[47] In joining forces, LACSA made a powerful ally.

The Municipal League made the formal request for action. The organization sent a letter to Mayor Owen C. McAleer in early February asking him to appoint a housing commission to "work for the eradication of slum conditions."[48] The league argued that the public's general welfare suffered from the "physical and moral evils arising from overcrowding." They also contended that the advent of slums was new. According to their letter, until 1900 housing problems were isolated to a few lodging houses and a few individual homes. They argued that the influx of "low-waged laborers" from Mexico and southern Europe had wrought the present conditions.

Although the league asked the mayor to allow the commission to investigate lodging houses and tenements, its letter focused on house courts "within a radius of a half a mile of the Plaza . . . aggregating an area of perhaps three city blocks." Despite believing that these dwellings were "better aired and better lighted than the eastern slum tenement," the league argued that the number of residents and the physical construction of the house courts negated any superiority. The courts were hazardous, according to the league's letter, because the "rotten boards, rusty tins and scraps of dirty cloth" that made up these dwellings were materials that "harbor[ed] disease." The league did not fault the health department for present conditions. Instead it argued that "despite of the utmost exertions of the Board of Health, they cannot be kept wholesome." The league was aware that there might be protest to change but argued that reformers in other cities had managed to enact reform that considered the "rights of property." The point of a commission would be to conduct further investigations and provide suggestions for reform. The appeal succeeded and, apparently without public or official dissent, the mayor appointed a commission on February 20, 1906.

When LACSA created its public health nursing program, it used public funds. The mayor's appointment of an advisory commission was a slightly different kind of quasi-public organization. The public health nurse's salary came from municipal funds but she reported to a private association. In this case, the commission received public authority to carry out its work but relied on private funds to do so. In the first two years, the Municipal League provided the commission with office space, library access, a stenographer, paper supplies, and a male inspector to document conditions. While the Municipal League kept its members informed through its monthly newsletter (no corresponding information is available for LACSA), the commission ultimately reported to a public authority.

Composed of a minister, physician, attorney, architect, and settlement worker, the housing commission reflected broad beliefs about what constituted public health. Each field brought a different view concerning the physical logistics as well as theoretical frameworks necessary for developing public health policy. Throughout its existence from 1910 to 1913, the commission's policies became increasingly divided into two related but distinct categories: regulation and education. This division reflected the perspective of the different groups involved. LACSA, for instance, tended to emphasize the power of instruction over legislation in their day-to-day work at the settlement. Like many middle-class women of the era, LACSA's settlement workers understood the necessity of structural amelioration but also believed that their efforts were doomed to fail unless they created an informed society. This gendered perception of reform became embodied in the 1913 merger of the housing commission within the city is health department.

The original members of the commission were LACSA member Mary Adair Veeder, physician Titian Coffey, the Reverend William Horace Day, attorney Elizabeth L. Kenney, and architect George E. Bergstrom.[49] None of these individuals were novices in their fields. A year later, the commission added two more representative fields, a capitalist and a plumber. The commission itself changed over the years in its scope of work and authority, but the commissioners themselves and these categories of representation remained relatively stable. Veeder served on the commission until 1917, the longest of the original five. She bridged the initial movement for reform to its official expression within the health department. In addition, unlike the other members of the commission, it appears to have been her only job. Her presence was the means by which LACSA continued to play an influential role in shaping housing reform in the city. Coffey presided as chairman until 1912, after which Bergstrom took over until 1919. Kenney remained until 1911. In addition, replacement appointees for the original five also remained fairly consistent. The Reverend Dana Bartlett and plumber Thomas Haverty were appointed in 1908 and continued their activities through 1922.

Initially the commission had two goals. The first was to engage in self-education on "the housing problem." They did so by investigating unsanitary housing conditions that existed throughout the United States. New York City's tenements provided the most obvious starting point. The New York Housing Act of 1867—the first of its kind in the nation—defined tenements as either single residences leased to three or more different families who shared cooking facilities or as two or more different families sharing toilet facilities.[50] Comparatively, the first legal definition of a house court, written in 1907 in Los Angeles, defined it as a super-structure within which "groups of three or more habitations us[ed] ground or facilities, or both in common."[51] The idea of common facilities was similar, but the house courts in Los Angeles were officially defined by the structures themselves, not the people within them. While different in official definition, the housing commissioners in Los Angeles recognized that, in substance, the house courts were "equivalent," and in some cases arguably worse, than the New York tenements.[52] Jacob Riis's descriptions of overcrowdedness, poor ventilation, and poor sanitation in New York City tenements closely resembled the types of public health problems that the Housing Commission of the City of Los Angeles discovered in the local house courts. However, since the commissioners did not find an exact replica of the house court in their studies, they declared themselves "forced to work out [their] own salvation."[53]

The commission's second goal was to survey housing conditions in the city. Although the commission wanted to investigate all forms of housing for the poor and working class, house courts became the immediate and dominant focus. These dwellings existed in the same immigrant neighborhoods within which LACSA already worked. That familiarity prompted the commissioners to focus on the courts even though only one percent of the population in Los Angeles in 1905 lived in these types of residences. At the same time, that percentage constituted a population of over two thousand.[54] In the opinion of the housing commissioners, the quality of the materials used to construct these buildings, their clustering, their lack of public utilities, and the conduct of the tenants made them untenable.

In the commission's initial surveys, it classified sixty-eight residential areas as house courts. These ranged from tracts of three houses to ones of almost seventy. They found one to eight people occupying single rooms, and ten to fifteen people living in smallish three-room houses. The commission contended that they frequently discovered families (husband, wife, and two to five children) living within a single room measuring seven by eight feet. They considered a house court on New High and Buena Vista Street a prime example of what offended them. Located just west of the old Chinatown—where Union Station is now located—and south of the Plaza, this house court ran 277 feet wide, had a depth of 161 feet, and, within this space, fifty-seven wooden structures of two to four rooms existed. The housing commission noted that "while toilet facilities existed, they were "too filthy for humans to use." They counted 170 official residents but argued that there were an uncalculated number of boarders who "crept" inside. The commissioners also reported similar conditions in the Utah Street court located just east of the Los Angeles River. They claimed that "between four and five hundred people, including children, lived in this area," but that landlords supplied them with only "seven faucets and eight toilets." Much to the reformers' chagrin, these toilets were unisex, resulting in what they argued was the "promiscuous" use of these facilities by "both sexes." Nationwide, progressive reformers tied the physicality of lavatory space to moral degeneracy.

The commission also associated architecture with disease. The commissioners' investigations showed that landlords often built house courts without constructing drainage. They noted that "it was a customary sight to see pools or gutters of stagnant, foul-smelling water, containing at times garbage, and attracting myriads of flies." Furthermore, the surface area was almost always unpaved, which meant in the winter the rains turned these surfaces into "veritable quagmires." In fact, the commission stressed that the conditions during the winter became so awful that they should be "better imagined than described." That the rainy season resulted in disastrous conditions was an ironic twist on the promotion of southern California's climate and a comment that female reformers had made on previous occasions. The housing commission also believed that the wooden construction of the house courts proved to be a "repository for dirt and germs" no matter what season.[55] Specifically, diphtheria, tuberculosis, and smallpox caused the commissioners concern.[56]

The commissioners delved into why these courts had come into being and why people stayed in them. They recognized that these neighborhoods were sometimes self-imposed, sometimes the result of prejudice, and sometimes a combination of the two forces. The commission believed that Russians wanted to live in close quarters: "The Russians are gregarious and have formed a 'Little Russia.' "[57] Comparatively, the commission argued that Mexican immigrants "[were] not anxious to live with their own race in a huddled district." Prejudice, according to the commission, kept Mexicans living in the house courts. In an annual report, the commission recounted the story of "Mrs. S.," a young Mexican woman, who lived in a two-room dwelling with her children. When the inspector came across her, "Mr. S." had recently died of tuberculosis within the home, and the oldest child, Feliz, a seven-year-old boy, had whooping cough. The inspector attempted to find a house for Mrs. S. with help from county authorities who would pay $10 a month for assistance. In trying to find a home outside the courts, Mrs. S. continually came up against a populace who bitterly opposed having Mexicans as neighbors. A survey of New York tenants on "tenement evils" that Robert W. DeForest and Lawrence Veiller included in their comprehensive 1903 manuscript on "The Tenement House Problem" offers some additional hints as to how local residents might have felt about their living conditions. In being asked about tenement conditions, tenants complained about the inadequacy of garbage facilities, the lack of room for storage, and the shoddy workmanship of the structures themselves.[58] Their comments resonated with Elsing's point in 1892: "The only reason why so many people put up with the numerous inconveniences of a tenement-house is simply that stern necessity compels them to live in this way."[59] Still, putting complaints aside, the testimonies also suggest that proximity to work, affordable rent, and access to familiar communities were equally important tenant concerns.

The commission as it was first crafted in 1906 could only record problems. It lacked the legal authority to impose correction. Furthermore, technically landlords had not violated any laws. Six months after its establishment, the commission was up for renewal. Despite its clear limitations, it faced opposition. Councilman Arthur D. Houghton was the commission's main opponent. He argued that "the whole thing was merely an attempt on the part of a few rich people to insult and make light of the poverty and misery of the poor of the city."[60] The *Los Angeles Times* responded by dubbing Houghton the "recall freak from the Sixth Ward." This was not the first time the *Times* had characterized Houghton in an unfavorable light. Two years earlier, he had won his position in the first recall election ever held in the city, which had been sparked by the city council's awarding the *Times* an exclusive printing contract. The Southern Pacific political machine in conjunction with the Typographical Union chose Houghton because he was representative of the skilled laborers residing in the sixth ward: Houghton was a member of the Electrical Workers Union.[61]

Based on Houghton's political appeal to the city's working classes, his objection to the housing commission's ability to inspect people's homes was not surprising. Emblematic of his populist stance, the *Times* quoted him as saying that he would advise property owners in his district to draw their revolvers if a housing commissioner attempted to enter their homes.[62] In retrospect, however, Houghton's apprehension proved unwarranted. His constituents had little to fear that the commission would scrutinize their homes. The Sixth Ward was the second largest ward in 1900 and contained the second largest number of native white residents, the fourth largest number of foreign whites, a small number of African Americans, and a very small number of Chinese.[63] According to a ward map from 1908 at the city's archives, the Sixth Ward was located southwest of downtown near Florence and Main, approximately thirty blocks south of LACSA's primary areas of concern. Consequently, the Sixth Ward did not attract the attention of housing reformers either demographically or geographically. The mayor renewed the commission over Houghton's objections. Still, his challenge might have had some impact. Although renewed, the mayor continued to limit the scope of the commission's authority.

Once renewed, the housing commission focused its efforts for the next five months on pressuring the city to adopt legislation to regulate house courts. In order to make their case, the commission utilized two competitive papers, the *Los Angeles Times* and *Los Angeles Express*, to publicize conditions to middle-class and working-class audiences.[64] In October 1906, the *Times* assisted the commission's quest for more authority by printing a front-page exposé on house-court conditions, complete with five photographs, which conveyed the opinion that house courts constituted a disease threat. Reiterating many of Stoddart's points from 1905, the *Times* contended, "Los Angeles has been so intent upon building her beautiful homes that she let her slums breed pestilence and crime without a word of protest." The *Times* also noted that these slums existed "just out of the vision of the tourists and suburbanites who daily pass by them in the Pasadena Cars." Similarly, the *Express* quoted the president of the commission, Titian Coffey, as saying that "it is no exaggeration to say that every person who passes even as near these places as the car takes them is exposed to contagion."

In addition to the newspapers, the commission engaged in a number of publicity engagements to drum up support. Coffey served as the spokesperson. On November 21, 1906, he reported on his work to the Los Angeles district of the California Federation of Women's Clubs at its sixth annual session.[65] The following day Coffey appeared before the board of health, where he produced "an elaborate map showing location of the Cholo and Mexican districts" and explained the commission's work. He also "presented draft of an ordinance" that would cover the house courts. In turn, the board thanked Coffey and recommended the proposed ordinance to the city council.[66] In turn the city council passed a "House Court Ordinance" on February 5, 1907. There was one objection on record: Councilman Clampitt did not vote for the ordinance, although there is no archival evidence indicating why.[67]

The House Court Ordinance defined house courts as well as stipulated certain building codes. The ordinance required owners to submit their building plans (the types of materials they wanted to use, the layout of the residences, and the location of sanitation and water supplies) to the city to receive approval before they could erect a new house court and to continue to lease those already in existence. The ordinance specified that water needed to drain off the houses, that windows needed to exist in living and sleeping quarters, that earthen floors were prohibited, that ceilings needed to be at least seven feet high, and that a certain ratio of toilets and hydrants exist per habitation and per man and woman. Also, the ordinance prescribed that 30 percent of the ground area was to be vacant to prevent overcrowding. The ordinance, however, did not specify how that percentage would be distributed. Consequently, according to the commission even after the passage of the ordinance, the courts still ended up with houses lined up in tight rows, "leaving rooms as dark, as sunless, as cheerless as in the worst type of cheap tenement."[68] Although the city passed this ordinance, it did not bestow police powers to the housing commission to enforce these rules. Instead, the responsibility for enforcing these regulations fell to the board of public works and the board of health. This division of power was similar to that in Buffalo, New York, a split which reformers there found impractical.[69] Whatever complaints local reformers might have had about this arrangement, however, they kept to themselves.

Although there is no public record of debate at the city council meeting where officials approved the House Court Ordinance, there were a variety of responses once it passed. The most immediate consequence was that the ordinance forced almost half of the house courts to close, leaving hundreds homeless. The Municipal League described scenes of confusion among the former tenants: "They do not understand what they have done that is wrong, and indeed the whole procedure is a complete mystery to them."[70] In addition, the league noted that the ordinance inadvertently replaced one public health problem with another: "They are settling in vacant lots and in the backyards in the poorer sections of town, where they will presently be ousted again by the Health Inspectors." The league downplayed the significance of this public health threat by arguing that "fortunately the weather is pleasant, and they are accustomed to out-of-door life, and the worst that can happen to them will scarcely be as bad as the conditions under which they have been living in the house courts." The league needed to make light of this chaos because the idea of unleashing a destitute and sickly mob on the city ran counter to its arguments about the benefits of housing reform for Los Angeles as a whole. Unfortunately, no documents appear to exist that would indicate how LACSA viewed the situation.

According to the commission, the property owners of the one-half of house courts that were left expressed little opposition to the ordinance. The commission recorded the installation of brick toilets, flush systems, water hoppers for hydrants to prevent leakage, windows, and floors. It estimated that landlords spent over $20,000 for these permanent improvements.[71] The commission believed that property owners complied when they recognized that these enhancements increased the value of their investments. According to the commissioners, repairs began right after the newspapers published the ordinance and before copies were distributed to landlords. Even after this initial reception the commission stated that compliance often occurred soon after either the department of public works or health department posted a notice of violation. Resistance was subject to a misdemeanor that carried a fine ranging from five to hundred dollars and five to fifty days in jail.

Still, the commission could not deny the fact that some landlords objected. It observed that some of the courts remained in substandard conditions and blamed it on the greed of property owners. Although they did not name the individual, the commissioners were frustrated that a wealthy Angeleno owned the house court on New High and Buena Vista Street: "The sad commentary upon such a plague spot being allowed to exist in the city is the fact that, backed by wealth and influence, this place has shown the least improvements of any of the courts in town."[72] The commission offered a stark contrast, describing how a "white-haired Señora," in making the necessary improvements, "mortgaged her property, and now takes pride in her remodeled and transformed adobes, buildings nearly hundred years old." That ethnic and gendered comparison reinforced the commission's belief that Mexicans and women were more sensitive to their issues.[73] Opposition, however, did not necessarily occur out of greed. In a rare explanation of landlord resistance, N. M. Melrose argued in a letter to the editor of the *Los Angeles Times* that he had complied with "every demand of this commission" until they "ordered me to tear off all cloth and paper put on by their order and substitute the heaviest canvas."[74] Exasperated, Melrose exclaimed, "Who ever heard of the 'heaviest canvas' or any kind of canvas being used for house lining?" Melrose disagreed with housing reformers' conception about what constituted a public health hazard.

The commission's desire to secure the support of women reflected its belief that education was as important as improving the edifices.[75] The members argued that the sanitary problems associated with the house courts originated inside the residences: "Filth and garbage is rarely carried from without in." They wanted to enter the interior of homes not only to inspect for faulty structures but what they saw as faulty living. Unlike their view of most owners, the commissioners believed that the "inhabitants of these courts, in many cases, transgress not viciously, but through ignorance." Furthermore, the commissioners viewed the interior of the home as a woman's domain; it was the wife and mother who was most often home alone during the day when the inspections were conducted. The commissioners found "that the women usually resent the investigation of a man inspector, no matter how tactfully carried [and that] they welcome into their homes and pour their troubles to one of their own sex." Based on eastern examples, and their own experiences with public health nursing, the commission determined that women were best equipped for the job of inspecting as well as education.[76] Their solution was to hire a female inspector, but they lacked the funds.

Once the city passed the house court ordinance, the commissioners began a new campaign to transform the commission from a purely advisory body to a regular city department. Jacob Riis inadvertently aided the commission's quest. Approximately a week before the ordinance passed in 1907, he again visited the city to talk about slums. This time he was not engaged in a lecture tour, but was in the area to rest for health reasons.[77] He gave only one organized talk, "The Battle with the Slums," which over thousand people attended. Producing a lecture that "was profusely illustrated with stereopticon views," Riis described his ongoing work in New York and the need for continued vigilance. According to Riis, in New York the tenement regulations provided for a sufficient allocation of air per person, but "it is not an uncommon thing, even now, to find thirteen people crowded into the space that, according to the law, should house three. The fight is going on all the time."[78] Nonetheless, Riis's descriptions of his work also provided a sense of optimism. He suggested that with diligence, permanent changes could be made. Although archival research yields no clues about his immediate impressions, in remarking on his journeys a few months later in the *Charities and the Commons*, Riis expressed his faith in western reformers' urban projects: "The West is the land of promise, of the future still, though frontiers have gone and the midday sun shines bright upon it, the land where they do things."[79]

The timing of Riis's visit appears coincidental, but the implications of his lecture were not. After his first visit there was agitation for a housing commission, after his second visit the commission pushed the city council and mayor to transform the commission into a regular and permanent part of city government, with its own police powers, regular budget, and the means to hire a female inspector. In order to effect this change, the commission conducted personal appeals to the mayor and to women's clubs for support.

In late July or early August, Housing Commissioner Coffey accompanied Mayor Arthur Harper through "the Russian and Cholo colonies in the Eighth Ward and followed for a distance the course of the river bed."[80] The *Los Angeles Times* reported Harper's impression: "I have lived here a long time . . . and I thought I knew Los Angeles. But I found conditions last week that have given me the nightmare ever since." It was after this that Harper asked the board of health to direct one of the health department's inspectors to work for the housing commission "for the purpose of bettering conditions in the tenement districts east of Main Street." The board agreed and "instruct[ed] Health Officer Powers to detail Inspector [Nicholas] Quierolo, who had been a sanitary inspector since December 1904, to work in the tenement district."[81] According to the *Times*, Quierolo's assistance was invaluable "for the housing work . . . because he speaks five languages."[82] Upon being appointed, Quierolo conducted a "systematic census of the congested districts" whose purpose was to then "issue notices to owners and occupants of these courts to comply with the city ordinances."[83] While this help did not go unappreciated, it did not fulfill the commission's true wish, which was to hire a female inspector.

A few months after Quierolo's appointment, the commission took its plea to the Ebell Club. On March 9, 1908, Coffey appeared before this woman's club, making an address, "Am I My Brother's Keeper."[84] He detailed house court conditions in Los Angeles and explained the purpose of the ordinance. While he reported improvement he also described areas where "men and women and little children are living in places worse than pig styes and little babies are coming into the world amid unspeakable squalor and filth. He also produced a map of a "new court" to be built "on sanitary lines."

As is evident from the Ebell, Coffey employed issues of women's health to effect change. Like any good muckraker, the commissioners attempted to shock sensibilities, especially female ones. In their reports, which were furnished to the larger women's clubs, the commissioners recounted stories to appeal to maternal instincts. They asked, "How can we expect under such fearfully unsanitary surroundings a woman will be safe from infection when called upon to become a mother?"[85] They continued by declaring, "Suffice it to say that frequently the women have gone through their agony lying on a pallet on the ground, not even having a bed of the most nondescript character. In one case twins were born when the mother lay upon an unhinged door supported by two wooden horses."[86]

Speaking to women's clubs was important not just for acquiring support based on women and family health issues but because many clubwomen were philanthropists. It was at the Ebell Club that it appears Coffey first raised the issue of model tenements. He "explained [to these clubwomen] what an advantageous investment such courts would be to the owners."[87] Although he did not mention the name Octavia Hill, her infamous philanthropic story—she bought and refurbished houses for the working classes of England in the mid-nineteenth century—could have served to inspire local women. In August, when the commission published its first report, it continued to discuss the promise of model house courts. Coffey argued that investors would receive 6 percent return on their investment. A few weeks after the report was published, Coffey apparently received interest from a "prominent Los Angeles capitalist."[88]

A year and a half later this publicity succeeded in helping the commission reach its goal. Without any recorded opposition, the city transformed the commission into a regular department in October 1908. Although still called the "housing commission," in its new arrangement it now had its own budget of $4,000 to save the city from a "scourge of dirt and disease."[89] According to its records, by legitimizing the commission's place as a regular department within city bureaucracy it was able to provoke landlords to invest "tens of thousands of dollars . . . in repairs and improvements" to their properties.[90] It some respects, however, it still remained a quasi-public institution. Private volunteers retained control over policy. In addition, the city structured the commission to maintain an interdependent relationship with the board of health and board of public works. The commission needed to rely on these other departments to take action in cases where building permits came into question, in responding to already existing building and sanitary codes, and in reacting to contagious diseases.

While limited in authority, the commission increased its staff to two inspectors, whose salaries took up over half the budget, at a hundred dollars each month. According to the commission, inspectors needed to possess "a good moral standing, tact, and common sense, a fair general education and some special qualifications, such as languages."[91] Once hired, the inspectors conducted from thirty to sixty weekly inspections of the house courts in addition to having personal interviews with the landlords.

The commission appointed a man and a woman and divided their duties based on their conception of male and female proclivities: "A man must know how to take measurements etc. and the woman must be a trained nurse to make her work effective."[92] The commission believed that nurses made the most desirable inspectors because they could identify unhealthy conditions and remedy them through instruction. Allegedly, male inspectors typically found it difficult to get past the woman guarding the door to her home, but the commissioners felt that "tactful" women inspectors could gain entry. As proof, the commission included testimonials: " 'Thank the Lord, it's a woman this time,' said the nice old Irish woman who for almost twenty years had never admitted an inspector. 'Do you think I would take a strange man through my bedrooms? They could not force me.' "[93] The commission argued that the "success" of the district nurses in Los Angeles attested "time and time again" to the advantages of employing a female inspector.[94]

The commission convinced a leading figure in the field of housing reform, Johanna Von Wagner, to accept the position as the first female housing inspector in Los Angeles.[95] She arrived in December 1908 after having worked the previous eleven years in Yonkers as the borough's first official female health inspector. She had an established reputation, having lectured on her work in the major eastern seaboard cities, in front of the State Board of Health of Massachusetts, and the International Women's Congress. Local residents could have known about Von Wagner and the role of women's clubs in advocating for her importance as early as 1902, when the *Los Angeles Times* reprinted an article from the *New York Tribune* detailing her work.[96] Von Wagner remained the Los Angeles housing commission's preeminent inspector until September 1912, whereupon she pursued similar work in other fields. Trained as a graduate nurse, she listed her qualifications as a "working knowledge of six languages . . . a special course in Domestic Science Dietetics, and the study of Public Hygiene." She found her knowledge of Russian especially useful because approximately four thousand of Russian immigrants lived within the house courts.

Von Wagner accepted the position in Los Angeles "realizing the necessity of preventive work in a city that has all the opportunities of becoming the metropolis of the West."[97] However, much like the city's response to Riis's infamous statement, "after a few months of inspection in this large but young city, [Von Wagner] was amazed at the extent of the housing problem and the peculiar difficulties to be overcome." Her studies demonstrated that New York City's immigrant working class actually lived in better housing than its Los Angeles peers. She noted that "there the average rent is $2 per room with conveniences in rooms. Here the most miserable rough, one-room shack with outdoor conveniences averages $3." Substandard conditions, according to Von Wagner, resulted in both moral and physical decay. She claimed that the "wretched

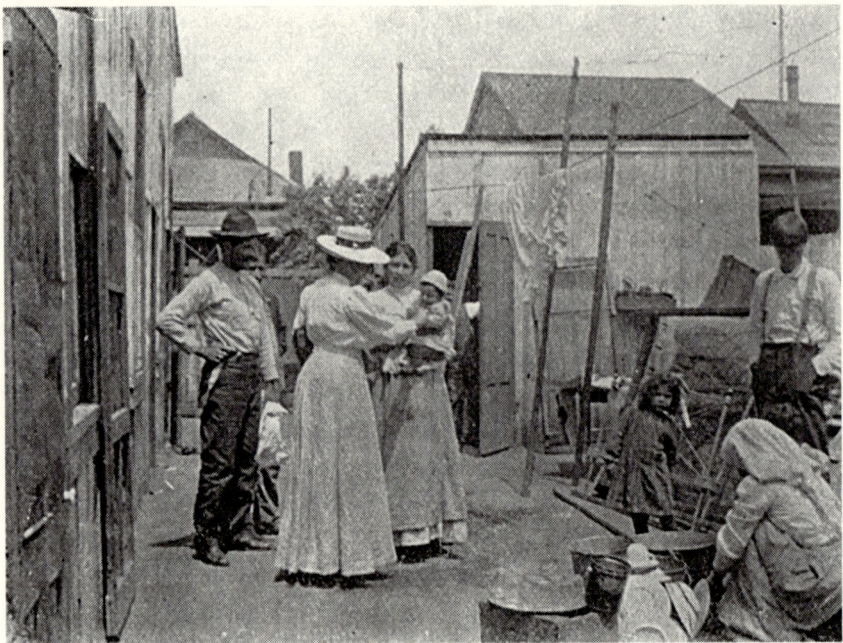

Figure 3 Johanna Von Wagner inspecting the house courts and its residents.
(Source: *Report of the Housing Commission of the City of Los* Angeles [1909–1910], 5. History and Special Collections Division, Louise M. Darling, Biomedical Library, UCLA)

habitations of the Chinese [in Los Angeles] have made it possible for them to pursue their opium habit." Nonetheless, Von Wagner believed that the climate in Los Angeles boasted the potential for a better way of life but warned that "the people in the West can not have better health than those in the East, unless they know . . . that bad food and strong drink are deadly."

Von Wagner noted several impediments to the commission's work. First, it was unable to communicate public health policy in a meaningful way to residents and landlords. Traditionally, once inspectors found a violation they posted a written notice informing the inhabitants and the property owner of the violation, but they only printed these notices in English. According to the *Los Angeles Times*, Von Wagner's effectiveness in New York stemmed from her ability to speak Russian and Italian.[98] Accordingly, the housing commission changed its strategy and created Spanish and Russian translations of its rules and contemplated creating ones in Italian and Slavonian. As a result, the commission found compliance increased.[99]

Despite success, the city's continued urbanization put limits on the commission's effectiveness. The problems associated with substandard housing began to exceed the commission's resources for response. The commissioners also believed that with the opening of the Owens River aqueduct and the Panama Canal that "Los Angeles [would] find itself a second New York."[100] The commission's reports from 1910 to 1913 indicated an alarming rise in substandard housing. According to the commission, rents were increasing out of proportion to income, forcing many laborers into overcrowded and unhealthy living conditions. The inspectors began to make night inspections and found, to their horror, men sleeping in chicken coops, and ten people sleeping in a room 10 feet by 10 feet. In order to respond to these conditions, the city increased the commission's annual appropriation to almost $7,000, which it used to hire an additional male and female inspector. But from 1912 to March 1913 alone, 409 house courts were created, bringing the total in Los Angeles to 621. Within these 621 house courts there were 3,671 dwellings containing 9,877 people.[101]

One way in which the commission responded to the increased construction was to intensify its calls for philanthropists to build model housing. Von Wagner spoke to the Liberal Club on July 18, 1909, arguing that what she had been "most struck with here is the indifference of the richer people to the need of less fortunate ones."[102] On January 18, 1910, Coffey, Von Wagner, and Bartlett appeared before the Charity Conference Committee. After receiving statistics from Coffey and personal testimony from Von Wagner, Bartlett "declared that he could see no reason why the people of the city should not unite in providing habitations for the poor in which they can live comfortably and well."[103]

Although these talks had an impact upon their audience, it was not necessarily the one the housing commission had in mind. The Friday Morning Club (FMC), for instance, asked the city to give it land upon which to create its own model village. The FMC did not want to share any responsibility for its creation or maintenance with the housing commission. "Mrs. Rundel" of the FMC, argued that "the work of the Housing Commission is so different from what we want to do . . . that we could not accept any arrangement that put it under that jurisdiction."[104] She drew a distinction between creating new housing versus renovating older structures. She argued, "I do not detract from the work of the housing commission . . . but the dissimilarity of purpose and method require absolutely separate management." Perhaps more encouraging to the housing commission was the formation of the Los Angeles Municipal Housing Commission (LAMHC).[105] Founded by John Randolph Haynes in 1912, it mimicked the Octavia Hill philanthropic model. Yet, after an initial wave of interest and an official action to incorporate, the LAMHC never sold enough stock to build or remodel any housing.

After five years of reform efforts, the commission had come to believe that the public health problem it faced was not embedded in the physical environment. The commission argued that the problem stemmed more directly from the customs and practices of tenants. Technically, a house court was only a group of three or more habitations using ground or facilities or both in common. The commission began to rehabilitate the term: "The house court plan is eminently suited to our climate and an ideal substitute for tenements.... In short, all classes are adopting them as being more desirable than apartments, more private and individual, yet less care than single houses and grounds."[106] They claimed that if built and kept properly, courts would maintain privacy, which, in their understanding, translated into a healthy moral and physical condition.[107] Consequently, the commissioners determined that the best course of action was to jettison their responsibility for conducting building inspections and concentrate fully on the educational aspects of housing reform as a public health issue. They decided to petition the city council to merge their program into the city health department and transfer their latter responsibilities to the board of public works. In this way, the two tenets of housing reform—regulation and education—would be maintained. Female reformers' request for legislation had been fulfilled, but their desire to conduct domestic education had been only partially realized.

In order to convince the public, Von Wagner's reports highlighted the impact of substandard housing on the health of women and children. Von Wagner informed readers that "the cry of this century is the cry of the children," and that "in some of the homes the faces of the sleeping babies are literally covered with flies."[108] She investigated the relationship between childhood mortality and the house courts and concluded that they were death traps. When Von Wagner inquired as to the number of children to whom women had given birth, she received numbers of eight, ten, and twelve. Yet when she calculated the number of children living in these residences, she found an average of between one and two. Von Wagner rhetorically asked: "Where are they?" She answered that "most of them are dead, a few living at home, and among the Mexicans many of the little ones in Institutions because there is no money to feed them."[109]

Von Wagner also recounted stories to persuade the public of the promise of reform. The use of female inspectors had been deemed crucial to conduct house-court inspections because they were supposed to be able to use their gender to garner influence among the occupants. Reformers did not consider their work as invasive. Instead, they drew a distinction between coercion and education, arguing that the first brought "enmity" while the other brought "co-operation."[110] The female inspector's role was to enforce the law, but it was also to identify areas of need and to assist occupants with securing appropriate aid. As an example, Von Wagner cited the case of one Mexican family who lived downtown near the gas works. Von Wagner noted that although the mother "was industrious . . . work as she might at the tub and in the house, Mrs. M.'s rooms and children were always dirty."[111] Von Wagner helped Mrs. M. move her family to the outskirts of the city. Von Wagner stated in her report that "these people are now responsible landowners with definite plans instead of wandering, irresponsible nomads, with neither interest nor hope in the future."

Not everyone, however, approved of this proposed split in duties. In July 1912, Milton W. Armstrong (a plumber) and Sarah J. Armstrong (his mother) of 974 El Molino Street submitted a petition to the city council arguing against amalgamating the housing and health departments.[112] In particular, their six-point objection called into question the ability of the health department to conduct this specialized work. In fact, there was no precedence for merging an ostensibly private program into the city's health department; LACSA was in the midst of a battle to get a nursing bureau accepted. The Armstrongs contended that "before the birth of the Commission the Health Department never educated its tenants how to keep their homes and premises clean, but kept the land-lords in hot water, which caused him to drive the tenants to other quarters." Beyond ineptness, they argued that a merger would disassemble the commission's successes: "To do away with the commission would mean to do away with the good work which has already been built up by them in the city."

Despite this expression of opposition, the agitation to merge the commission into the health department came to fruition on March 25, 1913. The Armstrongs were right about one thing: it appears that this action was unprecedented. The leader in these issues, New York, maintained a separate department within its city government to tend to the issues of the tenements. This was the same model Los Angeles originally had adopted. Yet, in 1913, the city council and the mayor in Los Angeles passed an ordinance to incorporate the organization in its entirety as a separate bureau with its own set of administrators within the health department. Reflecting its history and current composition, the ordinance stipulated that the commission consist of seven people, two of which needed to be women. This ensured female reformers a continued influence over public health policy related to housing.

Although there were no "nays" from the city council or any public objection voiced at the meeting, the transition did not go smoothly.[113] The ordinance empowered the chief health officer to appoint the housing commissioners, and Powers dragged his heels. While he offered no public statements for his resistance, this ordinance was a departure from the manner by which the health department had developed specializations. Typically, the city expanded the health department's authority without any oversight from volunteers. For instance, after passing an ordinance in 1907, the city authorized the health department to inspect hotels, lodging houses, apartment houses, and tenement houses. While Powers noted in his annual report of 1910 how difficult it was to execute this work in Los Angeles—he calculated that there were over two thousand of these spaces that needed to be inspected—he asked for more inspectors, not an adjunct advisory group to construct policy.[114] In response to Powers's reticence, the housing commission went ahead and held its regular meeting and declared it would keep doing so until Powers made his appointments.[115] Powers bowed to this pressure and subsequently appointed them as the new officials.

The new housing commission emphasized its social service aspects and no longer dealt with the details of construction, these instead becoming the purview of the building department. While limited in this respect, the scope of the new commission was enhanced. The commission was charged with inspecting house courts, tenements, lodging houses, and hotels, basically anything that could be construed as shelter. This fulfilled one of the commission's original goals. In addition, the commissioners were now considered assistant health commissioners and were granted the right to "exercise the power of regular police officers of the city of Los Angeles."[116]

Officials modified their strategies for housing reform once it was incorporated into the city's health department. Over the next decade, they changed the type of housing they deemed in need of amelioration. Jacob Riis's lecture had originally provoked women in Los Angeles to recognize the deplorable conditions in the house courts. Seven years later, another eastern reformer perceived a new housing issue before local female reformers did. John Ihdler, the field secretary of the National Housing Association, warned reformer Katherine Philips Edson in 1912 that "it is not your court houses which constitute the housing problem in Los Angeles, but cheap apartment houses."[117]

In 1906, Edson's cohorts in Los Angeles had responded to the squalid living conditions within the city by targeting house courts because they appeared to be the dominant form of shelter being constructed for the city's working-class families. Yet shortly after the privately controlled program had been grafted onto the health department, officials noticed that tenements were rapidly outpacing the house courts in number. (The housing bureau defined apartment houses as tenements.)[118] The bureau's statistics reflected this development. In 1914, house courts constituted 48 percent of all inspections and tenements 22 percent.[119] By the early 1920s, these figures were almost reversed. These numbers still did not completely explain why officials ceased to focus their attention on house courts because contractors still built a substantial quantity to house the rapid influx of new migrants flocking to the city. In 1922, the bureau recorded the presence of 1,508 new house courts, up from 317 the year before. However, the physical structure of these new house courts was vastly improved over their predecessors. Housing reformers in the 1920s no longer viewed house courts as symbols of blight. Instead, they understood them as contributing to making Los Angeles a "City of Homes."[120]

Related to the change in the type of structure considered ripe for housing reform, officials redefined the goals of housing inspection. Originally, female reformers believed that an essential element of housing reform was instruction in the etiquette of domestic hygiene. These women directed male inspectors to handle the habitations of single men—lodging houses, tenements, and hotels—because they deemed "education" an unachievable activity among that population. In contrast to their view of house courts, female reformers never believed that such residences could become homes. Middle-class women decided that only female inspectors should attend to the house courts because they believed that femininity was the key to influencing the wives and mothers who cared for these residences. In the face of a continually increasing workload, however, the new bureau determined that it could no longer justify this division of labor. In the 1920s, it abandoned the educational aspects of housing reform in favor of police fines and the condemnation of substandard housing. In addition, the structure of the bureau changed. In 1923, the health department combined the bureau of housing and the department's sanitation division together to form the Bureau of Housing and Sanitation. It appears at this point that the commissioners were eliminated and replaced with a single director. After the new charter in 1924, the new chief health officer, George Parrish, took the opportunity to further reorganize the health department. Under the Bureau of Housing and Sanitation, he added the work of restaurant, barber shop, and bakery inspection. As a result of these two acts, volunteer reformers no longer had any formal influence over housing issues and the focus on housing itself as a public health issue became attenuated.

While modified in many respects, a significant feature of female reformers' initial conception of housing reform still shaped policy. Officials remained concerned about house courts that were occupied predominantly by Mexicans. However, whereas housing reformers had blamed greedy landlords for dangerous conditions, they now increasingly faulted the tenants. In 1916, the housing bureau participated in two public exhibits, one at the Los Angeles High School for the Civic Center League and the other at the Robinson Building for the National Baby Week Show.[121] They included several dioramas, one of which was of a "typical Mexican house-court" complete with a female figurine. According to the health officials, "This exhibit showed exact miniatures of a Mexican home-made shack and a typical Mexican house-court with ugly surroundings." Claiming their model represented the "average style of architecture of the Mexican home," their depiction included "bad drainage, bad ventilation of rooms, defective screens, broken windows, improper disposal of garbage and refuse, and no provision for shade in the summer or family privacy." In comparison, they placed another three-dimensional scene of a "practical, up-to-date three room frame house" across the table. These visual images helped to confirm the belief that the Mexican population's living arrangements put the public's health at risk.[122] Consequently, public health officials contributed to a growing discourse that labeled Mexicans as a city "problem."[123]

Housing reform went through several different permutations from its inception after Jacob Riis's visit in 1905 to the establishment of a Bureau of Housing in the city health department in 1913. In 1906, Los Angeles not only admitted but also publicized that it had slums. Members of LACSA located the problem in house courts and succeeded in creating a government-sponsored commission to attend to the issue. At first, these women believed that both the physical structure of the house courts as well as the customs and behaviors of the inhabitants caused public health problems. Over time, housing reformers redefined the house court from a symbol of blight to a symbol of promise. The living practices of the immigrant inhabitants, however, remained suspect. In response, female reformers continued to believe that education was the solution to housing as a public health issue. In 1913, they merged this vision of public health policy for housing issues into the city's infrastructure and it remained so until the health department eliminated the commission in the 1920s, and with it women's direct influence over policy.

Chapter 3

Bovines, Babies, and Bacteriology
The Problems of Crafting Milk Reform

On May 28, 1912, Katherine Philips Edson took her seven-year-old son by the hand and headed for her local polling precinct. Women had recently won suffrage in California, and Edson went to exercise her new right. This was a special referendum election, and she needed to consider a number of very different issues. Should she support the creation of an Aqueduct Investigation Board? Should she allow the city to collect funds to erect a new city hall? On this day, the question on the ballot that interested her most was the one that she had played a role in crafting. It read: "Shall the ordinance providing for the tuberculin test to be applied to dairy cattle producing milk furnished to the City of Los Angeles, or its inhabitants, be adopted?" After casting her vote, she remained outside with her son at her side and attempted to persuade the electorate that they should vote in favor of the tuberculin ordinance because it protected the public, especially children, from tuberculosis. The *Los Angeles Herald* photographed her plea for pure milk and placed the photo on the front page of the evening edition. Much to Edson's dismay, however, the bill was resoundingly defeated.

Why did the public reject this effort at providing the city with pure milk? As the photograph illustrated, Edson used motherhood to influence voters. However, no one who participated in these debates displayed indifference to the law's possible impact on children. Instead, they differed in how they conceptualized the problem of supplying food for their families. Edson and other supporters of the law (mainly middle-class reformers, health officials, and physicians) characterized pure milk primarily as a technological difficulty, by which they meant the mechanical procedures for producing, packaging, and distributing milk. From their perspective, the use of scientific diagnostic tests to detect dangerous microbes was an integral part of this process, and Edson viewed tuberculin testing as the latest innovation in this field. Their opposition (a coalition of small dairy farmers represented by a socialist woman named Laura Locke) questioned whether tuberculin testing would in fact result in safer milk. They further stressed that the expense of implementing this new method of analysis threatened to drive small local producers out of business and thus raise the price of milk beyond what working-class families could really afford. While both sides concurred that the problem of bringing milk from the cow to the consumer was an important public health issue, they disagreed over whether the local state should be more concerned with supervising the system of production or worrying about the price of the product.

Foremost then, Los Angeles's battle over the tuberculin ordinance reveals how the general public, particularly women, attempted to reconcile the needs of their families with public health measures intended to protect the community. In this way, it is a story of consumer rights. At the same time, this episode demonstrates a lack of consensus over the meaning of those rights. Not surprisingly, class played an important role in shaping consumers' outlooks. Despite recent coalitions in the California suffrage movement that transcended class boundaries, women's power over the household purse had been a significant class-based partisan issue since the tariff debates of the 1880s.[1] When faced with questions of affordability, Los Angelenos in 1912 were divided on whether this law was truly in their families' best interests.

Unlike public health nursing and housing reform, general civic concern over ensuring the integrity of a community's milk supply was not a new health issue in 1912. Some of the earliest public health efforts throughout the nation in the nineteenth century focused on food safety, especially milk.[2] Consequently, when women became engaged in campaigns for pure milk in Los Angeles, they entered into an ongoing conversation among public health officials, physicians, and businessmen. At the same time, female reformers changed the nature of the debate. Reform-minded women employed science to justify their vision of an active municipal government but found their use of it as a political tool for public health action less effective then their use of sympathy.

Despite some continuity, a number of factors in 1912 set milk reform apart from nineteenth-century efforts. First, the sheer number of urban dwellers in the early twentieth century prompted the dairy industry to produce fluid milk, in addition to cheese and butter, for mass consumption. Scholars of geography and of rural history have studied the development of dairy as an industry with an emphasis on the Northeast and Midwest because these areas played a dominant role in its creation.³ The controversy in Los Angeles hints at some interesting similarities and contrasts. In particular, the "disappearance of the city cow" in turn-of-the-twentieth-century America symbolically marked a critical moment in a community's history: its transformation into a modern urban entity.⁴ Residents in Los Angeles aspiring to middle-class status viewed cows as an impediment. As the inhabitants living between Temple Street, Melrose Avenue, Vermont Avenue, and Michaeltorena Street argued, banishing cows would "accord [them the] same restrictions as other high class residential districts."⁵

At the time of the referendum, over 300,000 people lived in Los Angeles, making it the seventeenth most populous city in the United States. Yet it was also a community still in the process of purging its cows. In 1900, the federal census found almost two thousand cows living within Los Angeles, a number officials considered tremendous for a city with a population over 100,000.⁶ The city council eventually agreed and passed an ordinance in 1908 to limit the presence of these animals.⁷

Scant evidence exists to explain the reluctance by some toward expelling bovines, but Alice Stoll's petition to the city council in 1915 is informative. It suggests that even those who contested the presence of cows did not deny their potential importance for working-class family economies. In the late summer, Stoll, along with twenty-four other residents (fifteen of whom were women) living at the intersection between Ash, Aldama, and Avenue 56, petitioned the city council to amend Ordinance 23,660 "in such a way that it will not take away the income from the one who owns the cow, but will give to the other party an opportunity to receive some revenue from her property as well."⁸ According to the petition, Stoll's neighbor kept a cow from which "he claim[ed] an income of $300.00 a year."⁹ Stoll was attempting to "rent her flats" to defray the cost of maintaining her property that was "heavily encumbered." The triangular configuration of the city block caused a peculiar problem. To keep the cow away from his residence, the neighbor's heifer resided only thirty feet from Stoll's front yard. Making matters worse, Stoll lived downwind from "the stench and unsightly conditions." She had appealed her case to health officials, who allegedly told her that outside of rewriting the law, there was little they could do. Stoll argued that "ten minutes ... would be all that would be required to convince any one of you of the justice of my application for action." Without comment, however, the city did not take a stand. Instead, chief health officer Luther Milton Powers "informed the [city council's Public Welfare] Committee that he [would] see that the provisions of the ordinance [were] complied with," presumably referring to the sanitary conditions that offended Stoll's sensibilities and negatively influenced her business prospects.

Despite the cows' continued presence in certain areas of the city, health officials estimated that by 1912 only five hundred remained. Moreover, these bovines produced a very small portion of the 35,000 gallons of milk consumed each day. Instead, over 85 percent of the city's milk supply came from 1,279 retail dairies located roughly 30 to 40 miles beyond city limits.[10] Thus, although Los Angeles grudgingly moved its bovines outside of its borders, by the time of the referendum the geographical separation between producer and consumer raised concerns that resembled those of other major metropolises. The board of health attempted to regulate the quality of milk, sanitary conditions at dairies, and the transportation of milk. In doing so, health officials encountered resistance over issues of inspection, standards, and control.

Questions of sanitation initially arose over matters of human tampering as opposed to the proliferation of microscopic organisms. In the nineteenth century, health officials focused on practices of adding chalk, plaster of Paris, and magnesia to milk, which gave it an appearance of wholesome richness when it actually lacked any fat content. Similar to actions taken throughout the nation by many public health officials, in 1874 the Los Angeles city council prohibited the sale of milk that had been injected with chemicals or foreign substances. Yet it did not establish a means for enforcing that legislation until after the city established a permanent board of health in 1889. At that point, the board appointed an individual who was not a physician to work as both a meat and milk inspector to force compliance. A few years later the board separated this position into two distinct jobs. While the appointment of George Hood as milk inspector does not appear to have generated controversy, a fragment of evidence from 1901 suggests that there was some question as to his professional diligence.

Although archival records leave no leads as to the motivation for his action, on February 11, 1901, J. F. Stout filed a petition accusing Hood of being complicit in fraud.[11] According to his affidavit, thirty-five-year-old Stout was periodically employed by "one of the largest dairies distributing milk in the city of Los Angeles." He claimed that his employer instructed him to add "formaline, coloring matter, and water" to the milk. He also claimed that when preparing the wagon to transport the milk to the city, his employer told him to leave one can "of pure milk" untouched. Stout stated that this can was "known as and called the 'inspector can'; that said so-called 'inspector can' was regularly loaded into said wagon on each day, and was so placed for the purpose of being sampled by the milk inspector." Stout argued that the tainted milk could have been found every day, but that he "was never molested in any manner by the health authorities for indulgence in the practice of adulteration." The petition does not detail to whom he told his story, but the clerk indicated in pencil that the city deferred to take any action until Thursday morning at which point the city council took additional affidavits from Thomas Vestal and Guy Peterson. The details of their stories resemble Stout's but do not provide any greater illumination as to motivation or offer leads for further research. City council minutes indicate that Hood brought a lawyer, Bryon Oliver, to represent him to refute the charges. He was successful. After an afternoon session on the matter, the charges were dropped. While fragmentary, these petitions spoke to long-standing public perceptions of collusion between the health department and large dairy interests in the city.

While the health department would later portray their contact with local dairies as amicable, hearing cases of alleged violations related to milk production was a staple activity. A diversity of dairy owners, both men and women, appeared before the board on charges of noncompliance. Most often they pleaded their cases without counsel and reached mutually satisfactory conclusions; dairy farmers agreed to correct the offending issue, and the city allowed them to continue conducting their business. At times these confrontations became public. In 1899, the *Los Angeles Times* began reporting the names of dairies who failed at compliance.[12] Sometimes they published more than lists. In 1907, for instance, William Niles experienced a public castigation. Niles, "a local capitalist," accused the health inspectors of discrimination.[13] They charged him of selling milk from cows with "diseased udders." They also claimed that Niles had resisted all of their attempts to help him clean up his dairy. As these snippets indicate, fighting over pure milk raised issues about the rights of the small independent businessman, in this case the dairyman, and the limits that could be placed upon him by the state.

The rise of the germ theory at the end of the nineteenth century transformed definitions of purity. While inspection remained a constant, the ways in which the city determined safety standards began to change. In 1905, the board of health began to use bacteriology counts to measure purity. The city decided to inform dairies on a regular basis when they had exceeded a bacteriological count of 500,000. They also ordered the city's bacteriologist to "give as much time as possible to milk inspection."[14] But did dairy farmers and the public understand this new measure? The *Los Angeles Times* attempted to translate science for a public audience. The paper described a cubic centimeter as being "as much milk as will lie on the point of an ordinary table knife."[15] The *Times* also contended that there was a correlation between bacteriological counts and sanitation: "The Health Board has compared the results of their investigations with the microscopical tests and found that in almost ever instance where cattle pens and milk houses were in unsanitary condition the number of colonies in the milk was unusually high." Still, as scholars have shown, understanding that microbes caused disease did not resolve all questions related to transmission or drastically alter sanitary strategies.[16] Powers continued to depend on cooperative farmers to maintain conditions at the place of production, and he feared that the city's rapid urbanization would ultimately destroy these bonds.

Unlike previous accusations of complicity, concern over rising bacteriological counts led Hood into trouble. The board of health demoted Hood in 1909. The board "believed Hood [was] not aggressive enough in his work and that a change might be a profitable experiment."[17] They replaced Hood with his assistant, E. W. Hotchkiss. When the mayor asked Powers if this would have a positive impact, Powers expressed doubt. According to the *Los Angeles Times*, Powers "was not asked for further advice." Part of his skepticism might have stemmed from his acquaintance with the larger politics of milk production in Los Angeles.

While wanting to improve the milk supply, the mayor "made it plain that there must be 'nothing radical' that might cause a 'milk famine.'" His concern about the availability of milk was not singular. In 1900, for instance, the *Los Angeles Times* articulated public anxiety over milk supplies. The *Times* claimed that "cows do not do as well in milk during warm weather, while the demand increases."[18] Beyond seasonal variances, the mayor might have also feared retribution from milk dealers if he took too strenuous action against them.

The existence of large business interests raised the issue of price control. Rumors of "milk trusts" appeared periodically in the local press from 1902 to the 1930s.[19] The issue had such cultural resonance that some dairies used it as a marketing tool. Horlick's prominently displayed the header "Not in a Milk Trust" on its ads for its malted milk, and Crescent Creamery advertised that they were "independent of the milk trust."[20] Another company combined the issue of trust busting with bacteriology. St. Charles Cream argued that "the Milk trust is raising the price of milk—and the milk raises but little cream. Here is your only solution to the milk problem—St. Charles-in cans without the cow taste—pure, no germs, for babies and all sorts of use it is the best and safest."[21]

Yet the question was not simply one of consumer interests versus big businesses. Dairies large and small accused each other of engaging in unfair business practices. In 1902, for instance, the Dairymen's Union accused George Fry and H. S. Graul, owners of the Standard Milk Company, of undercutting prices. Fry and Graul did not own any cattle but purchased milk from dairies and sold it to consumers and retailers.[22]

Buying and reselling milk was a common business strategy. In 1907, Zenobia Palmyra Wilson, a widow with two children and a dairy entrepreneur, charged the Alpine Dairy Company of foul trade. Her story underscores the ways in which a variety of women used their role as mothers in the early twentieth century to influence public policy.[23] Although Wilson owned her own cows, she needed additional milk to make up for an insufficient supply. She attempted to purchase milk from Alpine but they rebuffed her request. According to her side of the story, they refused to sell her milk because she sold it at cheap rates. Frank F. Pellissier, a representative of the dairy, argued that he "did not know of any dairy being run by Mrs. Wilson and that no orders had been given not to sell her milk." In fact, he argued, the dairy did not have any milk to spare to sell to anyone other than its customers. According to the *Los Angeles Times*, the dairy supplied "over 3,000 families [in Los Angeles] as well as most of the hotels and restaurants." The *Times* was sympathetic to Wilson, allowing her to tell her side of the story: "I haven't got a husband to stand up for me, but I'll fight for myself and children. I'll give them a run. They'll see they can't drive me out of business." The *Times* described her as "plucky" and included a picture of her with her children. Approximately one week after her story appeared in the press, the Los Angeles Butter Board of Trade lowered milk prices in the city. In response, the Alpine Dairy Company claimed that Wilson had "cost [them] hundreds of dollars."

These doings sparked the interest of the mayor. Four days after lowering prices, in early February 1907, rumors of a "milk trust" prompted newly elected mayor Arthur C. Harper to summon Powers into his office and order him to investigate the issue. The local press supported Harper's inquiries. The *Los Angeles Herald* argued that milk prices were too high, and the *Los Angeles Times* named the Alpine Dairy Company as the culprit.[24] Even the federal government seemed interested. The day after the initial story broke, E. A. McDonald of the U.S. Department of Agriculture met with Powers and Harper to discuss dairy conditions in Los Angeles. According to the *Herald*, the timing was coincidental, but the *Times* put a more dramatic spin on the event reporting that "Secretary Kennedy almost dropped out of his official chair yesterday morning when a quiet appearing stranger entered the mayor's outer office and handed him a card."[25] McDonald met with Harper and Powers for an hour before spending the rest of the afternoon driving with Powers around the "outskirts of the city" visiting the dairies.

Yet, Harper's milk busting did not go any further. His advisers felt that "the most effective weapon [was] sharp inspection of milk and higher taxation of the wagons, if drastic measures [were] needed."[26] According to the *Times*, the problem "was not so much the stock as it was the cans that were watered."[27] Still, later that year when prices rose again, accusations reemerged about the existence of a milk trust. In response, the Los Angeles Creamery Company contended that milk had become more costly to produce.[28] Similarly, the Alpine Dairy suggested that rising costs resulted from a lack of pasturage. They argued that the expansion of the city had reduced the areas where dairy farms could exist.[29] Thus, dairy producers and health officials shared a perception that urbanization influenced the production of pure milk.

For health officials this concern led to increasing worries about safety in transportation. Two years prior to his demotion, in 1907, Hood submitted a special report to the board of health alerting them to the fact that the milk being shipped over the Pacific Electric Railway was "standing exposed to the rays of the sun without cover."[30] The board decided to send written notification to all companies shipping milk that they should "provide proper covering or sheds for the protection of the milk from the sun and heat at their respective stations where milk is received." If they heeded the request it was only temporary. In August 1909, the board asked Powers to "write Wells Fargo & Company that unless shipments of milk to Los Angeles from Buena Park Station and the cans were handled better shipments would be stopped."[31] Although the board singled out Wells Fargo as particularly culprit, it determined that most transportation companies paid "little or no attention" to shipments of milk. Moreover, not only were companies negligent but, in the board's assessment, their employees were overtly resistant to change: "In some cases they are insolent if requested to place the milk in a shady place."[32] Outside of making recommendations, however, there was little the board could do. As the board of health stated in 1910, "their efforts towards securing a sanitary milk supply for this city [were] being hampered by the fact that there [was] no jurisdiction over milk while it [was] in process of transportation by common carriers."[33] Local authorities could not regulate dairies that sat outside of the city's official political borders.

Frustrated but not defeated, the health department was ready to accept help from outside sources in its attempts to secure safe milk for city residents. The strategies public health officials had developed to cope with milk regulation shaped the discourse of reform. "Pure milk," for instance, remained the dominant terminology. Moreover, public health officials' long-term engagement with this issue meant that female reformers would have to engage in a well-established reform tradition. Still, women's articulation of the problem differed from male health officials and so would their solutions.

At the turn of the twentieth century, urban reformers were especially worried about the milk supply's impact on the health of infants and small children.[34] While the general public and the medical community agreed in theory that women's breast milk was the best food for infants, the practice of breastfeeding was in decline during this period.[35] Aware of the predicament of middle-class mothers, female reformers in Los Angeles used maternalism, an "ideology deeply rooted in long-standing cultural traditions that assumed a female prerogative in matters of children's welfare," to transform the question of milk reform into a women's issue.[36] Their heightened awareness of the dangers of urban living persuaded them to make pure milk an imperative public health matter. Moreover, women's enfranchisement in California in the fall of 1911 empowered them with the possibility of rendering their vision into law.

However, the pure milk debate in Los Angeles also suggests that female reformers understood and used alternative paths to maternalism in advocating for milk reform. Although Katherine Philips Edson used sympathy in campaigning for the tuberculin ordinance, she stressed science. At first glance this might appear to be an unusual tactic, especially since women at this time were successfully using maternalism to justify the creation of the federal Children's Bureau. Influential studies on culture and urban planning, however, document the emergence of an inextricable relationship between technological change and public health movements during this period. Although these works tend to either leave women on the sidelines or suggest that they were uninterested in using science as a strategy, new research indicates that women were as interested in using scientific solutions to justify an expanded role for government and citizen action as they were in offering maternalist arguments.[37]

Several emerging technologies were available to reformers: pasteurization, certification, and tuberculin testing. However, each of these approaches was controversial. Nathan Straus had demonstrated the benefits of pasteurized milk in 1897, when he cut the death rate in half for children at the Randall Island Infant Asylum in New York City.[38] Yet popular perception remained skeptical of the process and its purity. Along with the public, health officials nationwide believed that dairies pasteurized unsanitary milk to sell to unsuspecting consumers.[39] Also, pasteurization—heating milk at 145°F for 30 minutes and then rapidly cooling it to below 50°F—was not yet standardized and the equipment necessary for large-scale pasteurization was costly. Certified milk, raw milk that had been scrutinized in its production and distribution by an independent national organization known as the Medical Milk Commission, was only available in limited quantities and was very expensive.[40] The commission's stipulation that certified milk had to come from tuberculin-tested cows contributed to its scarcity. Tuberculin testing allegedly identified tuberculosis-diseased cows, but in the early twentieth century scientists disagreed about whether tuberculosis in cows could even be transmitted to humans through milk. Building upon this scientific uncertainty, dairymen questioned the efficacy of this test for protecting the public's health. Their intransigence also protected their investments.

Scholars of public health, the history of medicine, and women's studies have analyzed controversies over pasteurization, certification, and tuberculin testing as separate events and mainly as battles between health officials and dairymen.[41] The 1912 referendum came at a historical moment in which debates about these new strategies overlapped. In addition, while these disputes were not exceptional to Los Angeles, they were settled in a unique manner. By voting, Los Angelenos determined their own fate, whereas the courts decided the legitimacy of similar regulations in other cities.[42] Ironically, the residents of Los Angeles used a progressive political tool to prevent the implementation of another progressive reform. Ultimately, in the face of scientific disagreement, public health reformers who focused on sick cows instead of sick children failed to persuade a price-conscious audience to ratify their plans.

Katherine Philips Edson became interested in pure milk reform in late August 1909 when confronted by reformer Florence Kelley about the "milk situation" in Los Angeles.[43] Although Edson was a mother of three and her father, a physician, had supported the regulation of milk in Ohio, she claimed that she had never thought about the quality of Los Angeles's milk supply until Kelley raised the question. Born and raised in Ohio and schooled in opera singing, Edson had moved with her husband, a music teacher, to an almond ranch in Antelope Valley in 1891. They had hoped to raise enough money to relocate to Europe to continue their music studies. Edson was twenty-one. Eight years later, after giving birth to two children and failing to see their European plan come to fruition, the Edsons gave up farming and moved to the city. There they became immersed in the local arts community. Edson became a member of the Friday Morning Club (FMC), the oldest women's club in Los Angeles. The FMC provided the city's white middle-class women with a social milieu as well as a forum for political action. Edson's penchant for organizing quickly led her to become the club's secretary and then vice president in 1908. It was in this position that she met Kelley a year later.

Florence Kelley was a renowned expert on industrial-labor conditions.[44] In the 1890s, she had worked in Chicago's Hull House and led the Illinois legislature to pass protective laws for working-class women and children. Afterwards, she moved to New York City to head the National Consumers' League, an organization that used public pressure to create better working conditions for labor. Kelley briefly toured through California in August 1909, and Edson seized the opportunity to invite her to Los Angeles to address the Friday Morning Club. At the time, California's women were agitating for state suffrage. Kelley suggested that she be allowed to address the club members on this pressing topic. Sensing that her reputation preceded her, she also told Edson that if the members preferred that she speak on child labor and working women she would defer to their wishes.[45] While Kelley was best known for her interest in industrial health questions, she was deeply concerned about a variety of public health issues, especially infant mortality. During her childhood, Kelley had lost a number of siblings to infant diarrhea. Caused by consuming contaminated food, water, or milk, this disease frequently struck during the summer months when edibles spoiled quickly in the heat. Her later role as the chief spokesperson for the Sheppard-Towner Maternity and Infancy Act of 1920 perhaps best illustrates the intensity of her interest in the subject.

Kelley's busy schedule allowed her to visit the city for only two days in late August. She spent the night in between at Edson's residence. Over dinner, Kelley peppered Edson with questions about the "milk situation" in Los Angeles, but much to her embarrassment, Edson could not answer. Moreover, she did not know of any woman in Los Angeles who could.[46] Soon after Kelley departed, Edson embarked on a campaign to educate herself and the Friday Morning Club on the status of the city's milk supply. The measure on the ballot was the end result of her endeavors, although she never desired a public referendum on the matter.

Kelley had raised a public health issue that most of her contemporaries, Edson included, associated with crowded cities and a compromised food supply. In contrast, Los Angeles was sold on sunshine, space, and healthy living. By contemporary standards, however, Los Angeles was a bustling metropolis. Its population of over 300,000 made it the seventeenth most populous city in the United States in 1910, the year after Kelley's visit.

From Edson's perspective, urbanization and issues of health were directly related. In her opinion, this rapid urbanization had led to problems because "bread and water [were] no longer controlled by the woman in her home."[47] Nineteenth-century ideology charged women with the responsibility of managing the domestic household, but twentieth-century urbanization presented unique problems that inhibited women's administration.[48] In the turn-of-the-twentieth-century city, middle-class women did not directly produce the items necessary for their family's existence; they purchased them. Eventually, Edson advocated collective action by women to ensure that the goods they procured were safe for consumption. She asked, "How can a woman who wants to do the right thing by her babies stay at home and keep quiet while they drink impure milk?"[49] Her characterization echoed that of Milton J. Rosenau, the foremost American expert on milk reform in the Progressive Era, who compared the situation to that of a long river with many tributaries, carrying myriad possible pollutants, that connected the cow's udder to the consumer's mouth.[50]

Edson also came to the conclusion that "women of leisure class," like herself, needed to act as municipal housekeepers not only for themselves but for their "sisters . . . who [were] too busy supporting themselves and their families" to engage in such activities.[51]

While Kelley was the catalyst for Edson's interest, milk reform was developing into a major turn-of-the-century reform issue. Popular magazines published sixty-six articles on milk from 1905 to 1909 that described pure milk campaigns throughout the nation in addition to providing practical advice on how to maintain hygienic milk.[52] New statistics on infant mortality provided the impetus. In the 1880s, the United States Bureau of the Census began to compile mortality statistics. At the local level, New York City began investigating infant mortality rates in the late 1900s. A picture began to emerge that many found alarming. In 1910, the national infant mortality rate was 124 deaths per thousand live births compared to 106 in Great Britain.[53] Although poverty was a factor, infant mortality was an issue for women of all classes. Milk became a locus for blame. Unlike the traditional public health focus on dairies, middle-class women from across the nation concentrated on issues of access. In addition to trying to secure better milk for their own families, they also created milk depots to distribute a higher-quality product among the cities' poorer classes.

Yet Los Angeles enjoyed a lower infant mortality rate than the national average during this time. In 1907, New York's rate was 144 per thousand, in Los Angeles it was 112.[54] In 1911, the rate in Los Angeles dropped to 89.2 per thousand. Moreover, the infant mortality rate due to digestive diseases, the category that contaminated milk directly affected, also had decreased significantly from the mid-1900s when it accounted for 20 percent of all deaths for children under five. However, digestive disease still accounted for 11 percent of these deaths at the time of Edson's study and 14 percent for children between the ages of one and two. Judging by these statistics, Edson could reasonably conclude that the city's children were at risk.

After Kelley's departure, Edson began investigating the city's "milk situation." First, she visited Los Angeles's chief health officer, Luther Milton Powers, at his office and convinced him to give a lecture at the Friday Morning Club in early October. Perhaps not coincidentally, one week before his speech the *Los Angeles Times* printed an article about the relationship between infant mortality and impure milk, wherein it argued that since "some indiscreet scientist put a drop of milk on the slide under his microscope," it had become public knowledge even among the "low brows . . . that nice, innocent-looking white milk might be a whole storage warehouse full of germs."[55] The FMC responded to Powers's talk by creating a committee on public health and appointing Edson as its head. Using this new position, Edson sent questionnaires to all the dairies in the Los Angeles area that sold their milk in the city. She also informed them that the committee would soon post their bacterial scores in the FMC's bulletins as well as the local newspapers.

Health officials and Edson believed that bacterial counts indicated quality because the popularization of the germ theory lent credence to the idea that high levels of bacteria caused outbreaks of disease. Thus, her letter was a threat. Edson insinuated that women would not buy milk from poorly performing dairies. However, her first attempt at using science for reform did not go as she anticipated. It turned out that her consumers did not understand the significance of the figure. Edson discovered to her dismay that the public was "not conversant with the meaning or value of the bacterial count."[56] Germs and microbes were still abstract concepts to much of the public. This initial failure prompted Edson to pursue a second course of action: the promotion of legislation. If the public could not decipher what was in their best interests, Edson would construct an institutional method for protecting the public's health.

Starting afresh, Edson began a six-month campaign to verse herself in pure-milk legislation. She put herself on the mailing list of the Medical Milk Commission, the boards of health of New York, Rochester, and Minneapolis. She acquired monographs from the Nathan Straus Laboratory in New York and read Kenelm Winslow's recently published "The Production and Handling of Clean Milk, Including Practical Milk." She also conducted surprise inspections.[57] As Edson understood it, pure milk encompassed the absence of adulteration as well as germs. Judging by the popular press, her methods and opinion were in agreement with reform efforts throughout the United States. *Good Housekeeping*, for instance, printed three articles during Edson's period of research that posited a relationship between contaminated milk and infant mortality and emphasized women's agency in realizing a solution. Edson could have found inspiration and encouragement in stories entitled "The Portland Pure Milk War: The Story of a Victory Won by a City's Housewives," "What Any Woman's Club Can Do in Reforming the Milk Supply," and "Clean Milk at Moderate Cost."[58]

Edson determined that Los Angeles's milk regulations were very good but that Powers's ability to enforce them was not. Edson blamed the city's politicians, arguing that Powers was "seriously handicapped in his work by unsympathetic boards of health and city councils."[59] She felt that Powers's inability to appoint his own inspectors inhibited his effectiveness. In addition, she considered his staff inadequate.[60] Edson created an alliance with Powers and also moved for a newer, stricter ordinance regulating milk.

Edson reported her findings to the Friday Morning Club in June 1910. She appealed to the 1,121 members to take up this cause because she believed that the "milk problem [was] essentially a woman's problem."[61] She used a maternalist argument, suggesting to her audience that it was up to women to "protect and care for their homes," especially their children, whom she viewed as the "ultimate consumers." She assessed the problem as one of control and supervision. Edson felt that the "best dairymen were forced out of the business" because dairying did not yield a high profit for individual farmers. She contended that this had left the Los Angeles market in the control of those who were "ignorant, careless and utterly unfitted to run a dairy that [was] not a menace to public health."

In her presentation to the FMC, Edson focused on the issue of bovine tuberculosis. She told these clubwomen that many cows in the Los Angeles area were stricken with the disease. Edson based her opinion on the estimates made by the county veterinarian, Ward B. Rowland. He suggested to her that, by visible inspection alone, veterinarians would find that at least 10 percent of the cows producing the city's milk supply had tuberculosis. More importantly, Rowland said that twice that number would be found if these cows were given the tuberculin test, which he suggested was the most advanced method for detection.[62] Government officials and popular magazines supported his contention that the traditional method of diagnosis was inadequate.[63] In fact, as early as 1897, some physicians in Los Angeles had advocated to the city's board of health that the tuberculin test ought to be widely administered to identify and rid herds of tuberculosis-diseased cows.[64] Rowland's calculations were significant because Edson believed that scientists had proven that bovine tuberculosis could be transmitted to people through milk.

Was milk a conduit? For centuries, physicians had theorized that tuberculosis originated from domesticated cattle. More recently, scientists debated whether bovine and human tuberculosis were the same disease. Robert Koch's identification of the tubercle bacillus in 1882 did not settle these questions. Koch himself argued that slightly different bacilli caused the disease in each case. Consequently, he believed that a threat of transmission from cows to people was negligible, a belief that turned out to be erroneous. Scientists working for the United States Department of Agriculture had begun gathering information to dislodge this notion but, at the time of Edson's appeal, few physicians contested Koch's theory and correctly argued that bovine tuberculosis posed a threat to human health.[65]

Health officials looked to their milk supply for an answer. Public health officials had often traced epidemics of typhoid and diphtheria to contaminated milk as well as to unspecified diuretic diseases that disproportionately affected children. In 1903, for instance, the Los Angeles board of health thanked the health officer for his "efficient manner" in "hand[ling] the epidemic of diphtheria in connection with cases of that disease discovered at the Westlake Dairy."[66] Now, in addition to those diseases they began to believe that bovine tuberculosis was an important cause of infant mortality. The connection, however, between childhood mortality and bovine tuberculosis was tenuous. Studies did not consistently link exposure to bovine tuberculosis to the development of tuberculosis in humans. Although tuberculosis accounted for 17.5 percent of all deaths in the city of Los Angeles in 1911, it was not a major cause of infant mortality. Tuberculosis caused only 6 percent of all deaths for children under five, and there was no proven case of bovine tuberculosis transmission to a child in the Los Angeles area.[67]

Koch developed tuberculin, a substance derived from the tubercle bacillus, as a cure for tuberculosis in 1890. Based on the success of others in creating vaccinations from their discoveries, Koch believed that an exposure to a sterilized version of the microbe, tuberculin, could heal. According to health officials in Los Angeles, the bacillus was grown for several weeks in beef broth, then filtered, then boiled down to one-tenth its original volume, killing any active germs and then filtered again to remove them.[68] By the 1910s, however, physicians had discarded tuberculin as "the" remedy when many patients experienced adverse reactions and sometimes death. Still, its usefulness as a diagnostic test in humans and cattle seemed fruitful and, despite the risks, some sanitariums continued to prescribe small doses of tuberculin until the late 1920s.[69] Francis Marion Pottenger, head of the Pottenger sanatorium for the treatment of tuberculosis in Monrovia, California, for instance, advocated the use of tuberculin as a preventative. He thought that tuberculosis could only develop in a hospitable host and that tuberculin would create a hostile environment. Not surprisingly, he became a leading proponent of the Los Angeles tuberculin ordinance.[70]

Although the mayor and city council gave verbal support to Edson's cause, they at first remained reluctant to offer monetary support for tuberculin testing. Asked about Edson's report to the Friday Morning Club, councilman Robert Martin Lusk reportedly said, "God bless the clubwomen. I don't know what we'd do without them" because the council did not have the time to "hunt out such matters."[71] Lusk pointed out, however, that no legislative action could be taken until the board of health recommended it. Mayor George Alexander initially "snorted" at Edson's report, defended Powers's record, and downplayed the failures of Powers's subordinates. Alexander argued, "Well, they are doing better than they did."[72] He also informed his audience that Los Angeles had no authority over county dairies that supplied much of the city with milk. This was a common problem for municipalities. If Alexander kept up with current events, he would also have known that to take any action would incite the dairymen's ire. After Milwaukee passed a tuberculin ordinance in 1908, dairymen from the region immediately challenged it in court. They argued that the city had no right to set rules for businesses located outside of the city's political jurisdiction. This basic question of authority was not settled until 1913, the year after Los Angeles's election, when the United States Supreme Court in *Adams vs. City of Milwaukee* (228 U.S. 572) found in favor of the city health department. Acting diplomatically, Alexander assured clubwomen that he agreed with them that pure milk was an important issue but suggested that the FMC take their concerns to the state legislature.

Elsewhere in the city, Edson's address sparked action. The Los Angeles College Settlement Association (LACSA) created a milk depot to distribute certified milk for infants.[73] Moreover, the board of health began discussing new milk regulations within two weeks of her speech. Initially they desired tuberculin testing. On June 28, 1910, the board adopted a resolution stating that the "board of health is determined to inforce [sic] the tuberculin test in the near future and have an ordinance passed to this effect by the council."[74] Yet, in its final proposal, the board left the test off. Instead, the board proposed stricter sanitation laws and standards.[75] In this way, it planned to build on the types of work that the health department already practiced rather than implement radical change.

Angry at the omission of tuberculin testing, Edson and representatives of the California Federation of Women's Clubs quickly presented themselves in front of the board. They argued that Edson's report demonstrated "the necessity for immediately safeguarding the public health by eliminating the tuberculosis cows."[76] During the next year and a half, advocates collected support for a tuberculin ordinance, specifically the aid of the health department.

Although the city's health officials have left us no direct evidence that says exactly how they felt about Edson and her report, the department began to produce materials that expressed their concern over their ability to adequately protect the city's milk supply. For a city known for its oranges as far away as Europe, it was ironic that the transportation of the local milk supply was a major concern. According to the city's chief milk inspector, George Hart, Los Angeles's primary milk supply came from within 30 to 40 miles of the city. Dairymen transported this milk by steam trains, electric streetcars, or trucks, none of which provided refrigeration that would have kept dangerous microbes at bay. Only trains traveling long distances provided refrigerated transport.

Although keeping milk cool was not a unique issue, Hart believed that the West presented particular problems in this matter.[77] He contended that many eastern cities used ice, which was not readily available throughout the year. Whether Hart's perception matched reality is unclear. As late as 1918, only 41 percent of Chicago's milk supply was transported in refrigerated railcars.[78] Ice aside, cool milk was a problem.

The need to monitor an increasingly large territory created further problems. Although the city had increased the number of milk inspectors to nine by 1911, inadequate transportation stymied their efforts. Five inspectors used horses with buggies, two used motorcycles, and two had cars. Hart recommended increasing their salaries from $100 to $125 a month so that they would all be able to afford automobiles.[79] Even more problematic, according to the board of health, was the "laxity" on the part of some of the inspectors in carrying out their work.[80]

In addition to recognizing that milk regulation was quickly slipping from their control, some city health officials in Los Angeles agreed with Edson's contention that bovine tuberculosis was a critical issue for the city. One month before the city council adopted the tuberculin ordinance, the Los Angeles health department reported that in one local case where officials used the test they found 22 out of 54 cattle (40 percent) infected with tuberculosis. Probably because they did not want to create a panic, the department qualified their findings by stating that they did not consider it likely that they would find such high infection rates at all the dairies in the area.[81]

In joining Edson's movement for the tuberculin test, Los Angeles's health officials argued that this "progressive city" was falling behind its eastern and midwestern counterparts. In actuality, cities had just begun to institute ordinances for pasteurization and tuberculin testing. Moreover, when they did dairymen and milk dealers immediately contested these regulations in court. Much to the chagrin of health officials, their adversaries obtained injunctions. From Montclair, New Jersey, to Milwaukee, Wisconsin, the same scenario played itself out. In each case, it took years before the courts made their rulings. The issue before the courts was not the merits of the tests themselves but their applicability. Could cities regulate what was outside their political boundaries? The United States Supreme Court determined that they could in 1913, ending the controversy over Milwaukee's 1908 tuberculin ordinance. Local politics, however, convinced many municipal public health officials to avoid the issue for the next decade. In Chicago, for instance, city officials did not require tuberculin testing until 1926 even though the supreme court of Illinois ruled that they could in 1914.

Thus, under pressure from women's groups and health officials in Los Angeles, the city council and mayor approved a tuberculin ordinance on November 28, 1911. This made it unlawful to bring milk into the city unless it was obtained from cows that had not reacted to tuberculin. The board of health established one temporary loophole. Until January 1, 1915, milk from reacting cows could be distributed if it was pasteurized. This mirrored a Chicago ordinance from 1908, which required milk to be pasteurized unless it came from tuberculin-tested cows. However, the impact of Chicago's law was mitigated because it did not define pasteurization. To avoid this problem, the Los Angeles ordinance defined pasteurization as the heating of milk to 145 degrees Fahrenheit for twenty minutes and then immediately cooling it to 60 degrees.[82] This process destroyed dangerous microbes and prevented their recurrence. Based on the work of Straus, this appeared to be an effective strategy, but it also reinforced fears regarding the overall quality of pasteurized milk. Those who violated the ordinance faced a maximum fine of $500 or six months imprisonment or both.

Although the city council approved the measure unanimously, critics did not allow the vote to occur without vocalizing their objections.[83] Two months later they had gained enough signatures to file a petition with the city clerk to put the issue to a referendum, an option available to the residents of Los Angeles since 1903. The clerk set the election on the milk referendum for May 28, 1912. The question on the ballot read, "Shall the ordinance providing for the tuberculin test to be applied to dairy cattle producing milk furnished to the City of Los Angeles, or its inhabitants, be adopted?" Proponents and opponents argued over the scientific connection between tuberculosis, cows, milk, and children. They also disagreed about the nature of the test, precedents, and the impact this ordinance would have for dairy farmers and consumer wallets.

Edson led the fight to save her ordinance, and she drew support from local leaders in the medical profession as well as California clubwomen. The Friday Morning Club, Ebell Club, and the Los Angeles District Federation of Women's clubs lent their aid. Powers, along with physician Francis M. Pottenger, owner of the Pottenger sanatorium for the treatment of tuberculosis, represented the medical community. Together, leaders from these groups established the Pure Milk Campaign Committee to combat the United Milk Producers Association.

The United Milk Producers Association formed "for the protection of dairy cattle against the unscrupulous political doctors" and was composed of approximately two hundred small milk producers.[84] According to their calculations, they each owned about 14 cows and two-thirds of them rented their land. Their estimated earnings came to $2 a day after taking into account their rent and the prices for feed. If they had been subscribing to the major dairy trade journals of the time or the local *California Cultivator*, they would have known about the industry's general discontent with tuberculin testing. For instance, despite the *Cultivator*'s editor of the "Live Stock and Dairy Section," Mina E. Sherman, continual reassurance to readers about the test's safety, letters to the editor repeatedly asked for further clarification.[85] The Producers Association never stated that there was an explicit strategy in having a female leader, but Laura M. Locke became the association's primary spokesperson. Her appointment suggests that the local dairy lobby had the foresight to use a woman to make maternal and monetary appeals. S.W.A. Carver, president of the Crescent Creamery, and Lydia Gertrude Sobieski, president of the Milk Consumer's League, also spoke for the opposition.[86]

The prominence of female speakers for both sides explains why many viewed this battle as a women's issue despite public health officials' long history of milk regulation and the participation of both men and women in the campaigns for and against the ordinance. For instance, the *Los Angeles Examiner* argued that it was "women who first started the fight for pure milk."[87] Throughout these debates, Locke and Edson justified women's participation in shaping public affairs as an extension of women's roles as household managers. Political parties began paying attention to women's consumer power in the late nineteenth century, and Edson made similar arguments in the California suffrage campaign of 1911.[88] While in agreement on women's centrality to this political issue, Edson and Locke differed over its substantive impact on families. How they viewed the milk question was directly related to their personal experiences and political identities.

Although the dangers of an impure milk supply affected both working and middle-class families, examining Locke and Edson's biographical information is helpful for understanding how class shaped perceptions of the pure milk problem. Six years younger then Edson, Locke was born and raised in Iowa.[89] She moved to Los Angeles with her husband, Charles E. Locke, a high school teacher, in 1902. Like Edson, Locke was a mother, but in 1912 Locke's child was eighteen while Edson's youngest was seven. Despite their common experiences as wives, mothers, and migrants from the Midwest, they wound up as rivals. Why? While Edson had grown up the daughter of a reform-minded physician who took an active role in state politics on behalf of women's rights, Locke was the daughter of a disabled Civil War veteran. Locke put herself through school, at first earning a teaching degree before graduating from the Still College of Osteopathy in Des Moines. It appears that for each of these women the personal became political. In Locke's case, her overriding concern about the price of food reflected her working-class upbringing. For her part, Edson believed that women would choose a sense of health safety over money matters.

A major difference between the two women was their political affiliations. While Edson was a progressive, Locke was a socialist. Despite a strong coalition between progressives and socialists in the successful California suffrage campaign of 1911, the relationship between these two groups in the immediate aftermath did not prove to be as congenial. Until late in 1911, when two union members confessed to bombing the *Los Angeles Times* building causing several deaths, socialism had enjoyed a heyday of popular support in Los Angeles. Just before the McNamara brothers confessed, it looked as if socialist Job Harriman would win the mayor's seat. Historian Gayle Gullett's description of the mayoral election of 1911 suggests that socialist women felt betrayed by progressive women's choice of Good Government candidate and incumbent George Alexander, whose support of an antipicketing ordinance was instrumental in suppressing a burgeoning labor movement.[90] The referendum on the tuberculin ordinance came on the heels of this discord. Edson, however, continued to believe in the existence of cross-class interests and worked for protective labor legislation at the state level.

Additionally, although some socialist women in Los Angeles participated in Friday Morning Club activities, Locke's only membership was with the Women's City Club, which was formed in 1911 to battle for suffrage.[91] This organization was overtly political, although nonpartisan. Locke's political perspective and her position as an outsider to the Ebell and Friday Morning Club helps to explain her motives because there is no direct evidence that she had formal ties to the dairy industry. In addition, as an osteopath, she worked on the margins of the medical profession. Locke's main argument, however, was not health oriented. She focused on the ordinance's economic impact on working-class consumers and their children.

Edson and Locke employed a number of venues to sway voters. Both made personal appearances before various civic and social organizations. They also actively used the city's presses to publicize their positions. While newspapers might not have been their favorite source for persuading the public, they are the materials that have survived in the greatest number.[92] The *Los Angeles Municipal News*, a nonpartisan weekly newspaper, provided each group with equal column lengths to present their argument side-by-side. The *Los Angeles Examiner*, a pro-union paper that William Randolph Hearst had established to compete with the staunchly anti-union *Los Angeles Times*, printed extensive articles on the subject. The city's two other dailies, the *Times* and the *Los Angeles Herald*, published information on the milk ordinance debate, although not at as great in length as these other papers. Locke and Edson also made a last-minute appeal in an explicitly socialist paper, the *Los Angeles Citizen*, the day before the election. In addition to using these fairly typical modes of persuasion, each side took more aggressive measures. The Milk Producers Association mailed four circulars directly to people's homes while Edson put a tuberculosis-diseased cow, a questionable tactic, in the Broadway department store's front window to win support.

Although women were successfully using maternalism to argue for the formation of the federal Children's Bureau at this historical moment, infant mortality did not play a central role in Los Angeles's battle over the tuberculin test. Instead, maternalistic appeals to save the city's children appeared as occasional one-liners. The *Los Angeles Herald*, for instance, printed an editorial three days before the election with the captivating title, "Put the Baby above the Cow." Similarly, on May 20, 1910, Edson ended a journalistic appeal entitled, "Mrs. Edson Gives Reasons for Belief in Tuberculin Test" with the phrase "vote yes and save the babies." Yet neither the editorial nor Edson's article provided detailed statistical data linking childhood mortality to tuberculosis-laden milk in Los Angeles. Presumably this is because they did not have any to give. The only figure Edson could and did cite, that as many as four hundred children under age five died annually in California from tuberculosis-diseased milk, was a controversial one. Physicians did not agree about its accuracy, and reformers in California had not conducted any surveys that might have substantiated their claims. Without specific statistics, proponents could only make general statements about the welfare of children. Thus, instead of hinging their arguments on the power of a mother's maternal instinct, they turned to an alternate discourse: science. Unlike maternalism, however, science was not viewed as intuitive knowledge. Consequently, the Pure Milk Campaign Committee spent its time constantly explaining the biology, chemistry, and bacteriology involved while opponents focused on questions of economics.

The most frequent question debated was whether tuberculosis could be transmitted from cows to people. The tuberculin test demonstrated whether or not a cow might be infected but not whether this infection was transmittable. Edson and a host of physicians correctly assumed this to be the case. In response, the United Milk Producers Association argued that the ordinance was an attempt by law "to enforce conformity to medical dogmas."[93] They also published a list in the *Municipal News* under the title "Beware When Doctors Disagree" of physicians in Los Angeles who either believed that the tuberculin test needed more experimentation before its usefulness could be guaranteed or who believed that it was of no value for public health efforts.[94] Although a few of these physicians later claimed that their position had been falsely reported, the existence of this list illustrated that doctors were divided on the question of the safety and necessity of tuberculin testing. Edson attempted to persuade the majority of the 568 registered members of the Los Angeles County Medical Society to take a stand.[95] She appeared before the organization on March 1, 1912, and followed up with a written plea in their local trade journal, the *Southern California Practitioner*. In her support, chief milk inspector Hart, chief health officer Powers, and sanatorium director Pottenger all spoke on the topic before the association in the three months prior to the election.[96] These repeated appeals suggest that the members remained undecided on the subject. Moreover, while Powers appeared in person before his colleagues, his name was suspiciously absent in press reports on the battle being waged. Despite the want of direct evidence as to his motives, it is reasonable to conclude that the division among the medical community would have influenced his degree of public involvement.

Why were physicians divided? One medical issue debated in the Los Angeles presses was an ambiguous statement made by Koch at the International Medical Congress held in Washington in 1908. Koch estimated that "eleven-twelfths" of all tuberculosis deaths were from pulmonary tuberculosis. What about the remaining one-twelfth? Pottenger interpreted Koch's statement to mean that the remainder came from contaminated milk and, consequently, estimated that four hundred out of the five thousand annual deaths from tuberculosis in California were the result of infected milk. While Pottenger's calculations might have been questionable, subsequent epidemiological studies proved the connection between the ingestion of milk from infected cows with the development of tuberculosis in humans. The United Milk Producers Association told the public that Pottenger had "grossly misquoted Koch." They argued that the "one-twelfth" not caused by the pulmonary form of the disease was caused by all other forms, of which bovine tuberculosis formed only a minuscule percentage. Pottenger's only defense was to argue that his was the greater authority since he had actually been present at the meeting where Koch made the statement and therefore knew Koch's "attitude."[97]

Given the pedantic nature of these battles, the words of Manly Bason, secretary of the Producers Association, probably had more resonance for the average layperson. He asked: "If milk was killing off babies as the health commissioners say, why don't it happen to the dairymen? Did you ever see a sickly looking dairyman? No, they are all strong, and their children are also."[98] If the public could not trust physicians to agree on whether cows could transmit their sicknesses to humans, could they trust in the safety of the tuberculin serum?

Opponents to the ordinance argued that tuberculin was the "toxic liquor of tuberculosis," suggesting that it was poisonous.[99] Their characterization was reflected in at least one letter to the editor of the *Los Angeles Examiner*, when a local piano tuner asked how the public "could relish milk from cattle when they know that tuberculosis germs have been pumped into them."[100] He further stated that he would prohibit his family from buying milk from the area if the ordinance was passed. In response, the Pure Milk Campaign attempted to reassure the public that the process of creating tuberculin "completely kill[ed] off all germ life," and that the supposed danger was "mere bug-a-boo."[101] The piano tuner's objection, however, suggests that although the germ theory had been accepted into popular culture, the finer points of science had been lost in that translation.

In the midst of questioning the medical issues involved, the United Milk Producers Association attacked the ordinance because it allowed for pasteurization. If a cow reacted to the test, its milk could be sold in the city if it was pasteurized. The association called this provision "monstrously stupid." They asserted that it sanctioned the sale of diseased milk. "Clean milk from healthy cows, not pasteurized milk from diseased cows" was their slogan.[102] Opponents to the ordinance contended that the milk rather than the cow was the issue, and therefore the milk not the cows should be tested. Thus, they advocated a return to traditional public health tactics where health officials traveled to dairies to examine the cows and their environs. Proponents had a difficult time countering these arguments because of their own doubts about pasteurization as well as their faith in sanitation. Edson and Hart, for instance, both viewed pasteurization as a temporary solution until certified milk could be made affordable to all.

What precedents could both sides look to for support? Opponents claimed that every state that had tried a compulsory law for tuberculin testing had elected to discard the measure. Illinois was the most cited example because Chicago had recently passed a similar milk ordinance. According to the United Milk Producers Association, the Chicago health commissioner who engineered the original ordinance regretted the decision. In addition, Illinois not only repealed its own tuberculin law in 1911 but also passed a measure prohibiting any city in the state from requiring the test.[103] The dairymen also cited the repeal of similar legislation in Massachusetts, Maine, Wisconsin, and even in Belgium and Germany. Pottenger replied, "Where it has been discarded it has usually been due to trickery."[104] In a boosteric appeal, supporters contended that if Los Angeles did not adopt the tuberculin test it would be "going backward and confessing our city far behind many of the east."[105]

Related to the question of precedent, the final disagreement was over the impact the ordinance would have on the city's milk supply. The United Milk Producers cited the case of Washington, D.C., where they claimed a similar measure created a milk famine by raising the price of milk until the law was suspended. In Los Angeles, opponents of the ordinance contended that the milk supply was already short. They believed that this law would only drive more small dairymen out of business, rendering "milk still scarcer and still higher in price."[106] Locke estimated that about one-fifth of the city's milk supply came from small independent dairymen who lived close enough to the city to market their own milk. They also sold the majority of the city's nonpasteurized milk. She argued that the next possible area from which to obtain milk was 250 miles away and that the freight charges would increase the price of milk substantially for the consumer. The fact that the longer ride might have provided refrigeration, protecting the milk, was not an issue that Locke addressed. Instead, Locke concentrated on the fact that the ordinance would "raise the price of milk to such a point that poor people could not afford to buy it at all." Wielding maternalism, she added that "of course, that would do away with the danger from cow tuberculosis for the poor children."[107]

Reflecting her socialist philosophy, Locke recommended the creation of a municipally owned and managed dairy to supply clean milk for the city's children. She believed that the city could then implement the test as well as check the cattle for other diseases carried in milk, which had proven to be much more prevalent. She argued that "this would protect the children not only from what little danger there might be from tuberculosis, but also from all other diseases which might be carried in the milk, and which cause 600 deaths where cow tuberculosis causes one."[108] She believed that the small dairymen could sell directly to the city, bypassing large business and transfer the risk for financial loss to the city. Locke appealed to the public to vote against the ordinance "unless you want to place the city absolutely under the control of the big dairymen and pay increased price for your milk to secure protection which does not protect against a danger which is very slight." Proponents of the ordinance asked the public to dismiss Locke's contentions as "clever subterfuges to delude you into the belief that you would be doing yourself an injury by voting for the tuberculin test," and asserting that "there is absolutely no truth in those statements."[109]

As the election date drew closer, the barbs became sharper on both sides. The *Los Angeles Examiner* described how "acrimonious accusations and recriminations are being bandied; both proponents and opponents are quoting the same authorities to sustain their views; one libel suit is threatened; the whole serving to befog the issue."[110] Because members of the United Milk Producers Association did not sign their treatises at first, their adversaries accused them of cowardice and dishonesty. Pottenger wrote, "It is easy to misquote scientific men of standing and give garbled reports of what they have said, if no one stands responsible for such misrepresentations."[111] He implied that any person who agreed with the association must be a fool: "Certainly thinking people will not accept the statements of such irresponsibles any more than they would fake patent medicine advertisements." Ultimately, Pottenger beseeched the public to dismiss the opposition: "Your interest—the interest in the conservation of your health—in protecting the life of your child, are not factors in their campaign. It is simply greed, greed, greed, your welfare comes last!" Locke continued her appeal to the working classes' common sense, stating that "you would hardly call them 'rich milk dealers,' would you, or call it 'organized greed,' when men are trying to secure a wage at $2.00 per day?"[112]

According to the *Examiner*, this debate was one of the most "heated and closely contested non-political election" issues in the city's history. Telephone calls to the health department increased just prior to the election.[113] At one meeting on May 23 at the Alembic Club, approximately two hundred persons attended to watch Edson and Locke debate the issue face-to-face.[114] Yet, in the days before the election, Edson and the Pure Milk Campaign Committee believed that they had won the public's support. They secured the endorsement of leading major newspapers.[115] The *Herald*, for instance, asked the public to "put the baby above the cow," and included testimonials from local religious and medical authorities. Advocates also seemed to find favor among the city's church congregations. The *Herald* reported that they rejoiced when the ministerial union voted unanimously over the objections of Sobieski to endorse the ordinance.[116] According to the *Examiner*, Edson was "confident their fight [was] won" a week prior to the election.[117] Still, advocates employed "prominent women to distribute literature in all the downtown stores."[118] This strategy indicated that they believed that women constituted their voter base.

Edson and her colleagues were in for a surprise. The public rejected the tuberculin ordinance 18,883 to 13,899, a difference of 5,000 votes. Across the city, 116 of 154 precincts voted against the ordinance.[119] The *Times* reported, "The death of the measure was taken much to heart by its advocates."[120] The editors of the *Southern California Practitioner*, the medical journal of local physicians, stated that the outcome was "such sad commentary on the intelligence and esthetics of the voters."[121] After its loss, the *Municipal News*'s editor felt duped because he found evidence that the opponents had falsified names of physicians who were in doubt of the usefulness of the test. Belying the paper's supposedly nonpartisan character, the *Municipal News* declared that it had "trusted too much." The editor suggested that although the paper still believed in "an uncensored discussion of public questions, we must take precaution in the future discussion to protect individual citizens being put to use by too energetic partisans."[122]

The advocates blamed the loss on two things. First, while they had pursued an active campaign prior to the election, even placarding the city with "striking posters," they believed that they had been outmaneuvered on the day of the election. According to the *Examiner*, "It was not even conjectured, however, that the dairymen had gone to the expense of hiring men to stand at each polling place to distribute literature to all voters." As quickly as this was learned, the women's clubs began to make a "systematic canvass of the precincts" but apparently it was too late.[123] Second, the Pure Milk Campaign Committee declared that it had been outfinanced. In total, Hart later declared, the opposition to the ordinance spent $20,000 to win.[124]

Although defeated, the referendum did not immediately quash debates over pure milk. Instead, it seemed to intensify divisions between dairy farmers and health officials. Two years after the controversial referendum in Los Angeles, state assemblyman J. W. Guiberson of Kings County introduced a bill to address public concerns about milk safety. Located in the Central Valley, Kings County was and still is an agricultural community. Guiberson proposed the formation of a five-person commission in every city, consisting of the health officer, a physician, a veterinarian, and two men with dairy interests to supervise each locale's milk supply. The commission could order the tuberculin test for any cow it believed was tubercular but only if it first discovered the presence of the tubercle bacillus in the milk, a time-consuming task. Edson characterized the bill as "pernicious" because of this very selective application of the tuberculin test, and Governor Hiram Johnson vetoed it.[125] Dairymen throughout California retaliated with a petition to have Johnson recalled but failed.[126]

After the United States Supreme Court decision in 1913 that determined that city health officials had the right to stipulate policies related to the quality of their milk supply whether or not the milk was produced within city limits, Californians reached a compromise. The state legislature ordered dairy farms that sold raw milk to administer tuberculin tests and accommodated dairy interests by delaying the law's implementation until the late fall of 1916. After the debacle in Los Angeles, however, health officials in Los Angeles were uncertain that the dairymen would cooperate and decided to "resort" to "moral suasion."[127] They began holding "milk contests" and secured the aid of Lulu H. Peters, chairman of the public health committee of the California

Federation of Women's Clubs and a physician, to conduct a major publicity campaign to appeal to the public. By the end of the decade, the health department reported a "rapid increase of improvement" in the quality of the city's milk supply related to these efforts.[128]

As for Edson, the defeat did not prove detrimental to her career. At the same time that she had conducted her milk investigations, she had also campaigned vigorously for Hiram Johnson's gubernatorial campaign in 1910. This earned her a position in Johnson's administration as a deputy inspector for the California Bureau of Labor Statistics in 1912. Working at the state level, she turned her attentions to women's labor conditions in the fruit, fish, and vegetable canneries and worked for a minimum-wage law for women and children that passed in 1913. She was, however, still resentful about her failed reform. In 1914 she wrote to Hiram Johnson about an interview that appeared in the Hearst papers in Los Angeles from Nathan Straus. He had admonished the city for having a bad milk supply that he claimed caused five times as many infant deaths as in New York City. Edson wrote, "It is a shocking thing if it is true, but I don't believe it. I am glad to have them scared to death, though. They deserve it the way they voted."[129]

Why did the public reject this attempt to expand the city's ability to provide pure milk for the city? First, the outcome of the election suggests that Locke's focus on economics was more compelling than Edson and her cohorts' repeated attempts to explain the scientific validity of the test. When faced with the option of siding with the middle-class woman and her controversial scientific data or the working-class woman who spoke about stretching the family budget, it appears that Los Angelenos picked the latter. Still, the use of science in this debate demonstrates that Edson understood that there were alternative political tools available to women other than maternalism. Perhaps less contentious scientific evidence would have made Edson's case more persuasive. Women's postsuffrage movements in California for passing protective legislation for female wage laborers and advancing women's legal rights would make use of both maternalist arguments and expert evidence. Thus, the concept of the woman as expert was not lost, but her data needed to be more secure.

Chapter 4

Delivering the City's Children
Midwives and Municipal Maternity Programs

The newly formed Division of Obstetrics of the Los Angeles city health department chose two photographs to represent their work in 1916. They entitled one "Before arrival of Maternity Service Physician and Nurse" and the other "After arrival of Maternity Service Physician and Nurse." In the first, a Mexican woman, with almost a half-smile on her face, sits calmly at the edge of a disheveled bed. In the second the same woman is prone, covered by a white sheet and a nurse, recognizable by her white uniform, leans over the expectant mother. A table has been placed next to the bed, on top of which are white surgical bowls and instruments. A white curtain hangs on a wall and another curtain separates this birth chamber from the other rooms in the house. Both nurse and patient await the physician. The photographs tell the story of the city's endeavors to assure the ascendancy of modern medicine. They also reveal a counternarrative; this woman expected to give birth at home.[1]

    At the height of a movement in the United States to regulate midwifery, health officials in the city of Los Angeles devised an unusual plan for doing so: they put the city itself in the midwifery business. At the same time that health officials in Los Angeles enacted traditional regulatory legislation to deal with the "midwife problem," they also established a Division of Obstetrics within the city's health department to provide prenatal and postnatal care for working-class immigrants. The city's version of this care was taken, however, in large part from the practice of the very midwives the city sought to supplant. Though historians have documented how, from the mid-nineteenth century on, the increasing transfer of medical care from the home to the hospital played a key role in the medicalization of birth and the resulting displacement of the midwife by the

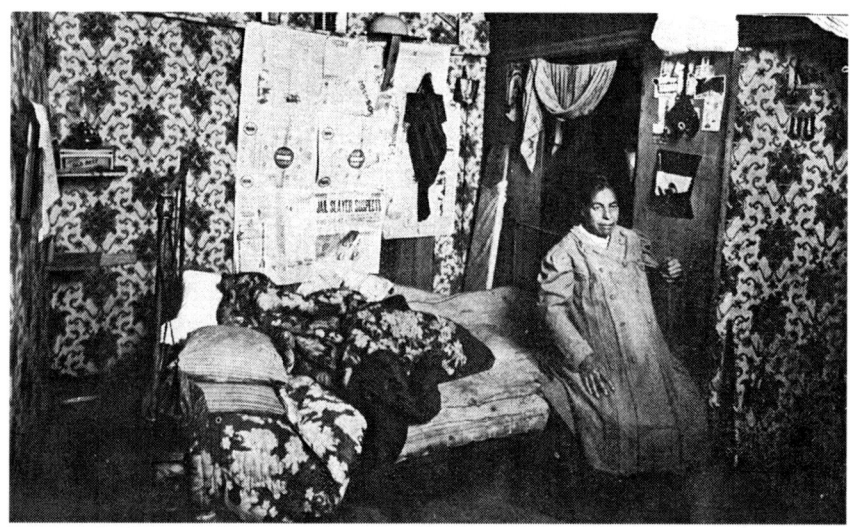

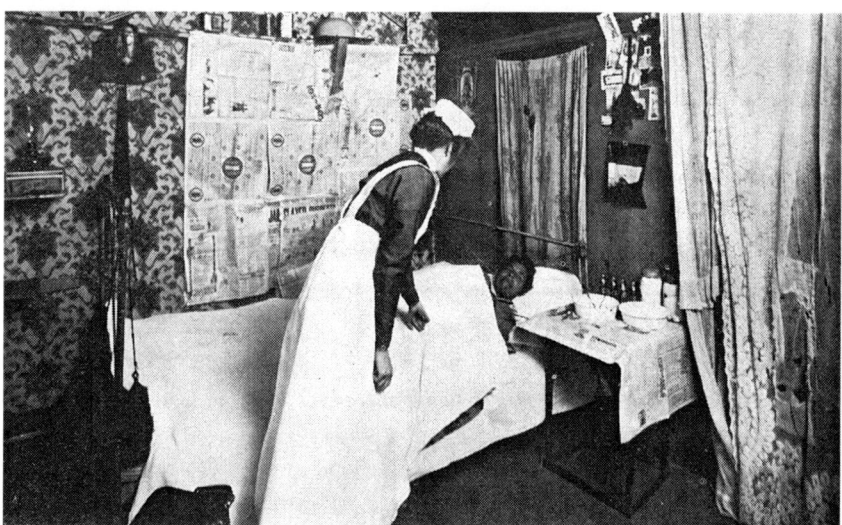

Figures 4 and 5 By posing its employees and patients, the city archived its sensibilities toward bringing modern medicine into people's homes.
(Source: *Annual Report of the Department of Health of the City of Los Angeles* [1916], History and Special Collections Division, Louise M. Darling, Biomedical Library, UCLA)

physician, in Los Angeles, unlike maternity dispensaries of other municipalities, the city provided physicians to attend home births.[2] Public health officials in Los Angeles believed that offering women biweekly exams throughout their pregnancy, physician-supervised births, and nurses' assistance at home for the following ten days corresponded to the care midwives typically rendered. Thus, rather than trying to move the delivery room out of the home, Los Angeles moved physicians in.

The city's program reflected changing social contours of twentieth-century medicine. Significantly, physicians were increasingly taking control of the birthing process for women of all classes. Yet, the more unusual features of the Los Angeles strategy serve to show that it was not the sole creation of physicians or city officials. Mostly white-middle-class female reformers had begun to shape the city's childbirth-related programs a decade earlier. These reformers, whose motives were often a direct result of a highly racialized consciousness, worked together with city officials and physicians to provide women in Los Angeles with the types of care they believed were in the best interest of maternal and infant health. They had already formed a general public health nursing program, worked to reform housing, and attempted to influence the regulation of milk. Developing medical services that focused on birth took the process of bringing municipal medical care into the home one step further. For various reasons, public health officials and female reformers never succeeded in their goal of ridding Los Angeles of midwifery. In fact, in attempting to undermine midwives' authority, the city broadly expanded its public health services in ways that mimicked the art of midwifery. Female reformers and city officials discovered they needed to bend to the will of the women they sought to treat if they were to have any success.

In looking at the role reformers played, it must be stressed that the debate over the "midwife problem" extended beyond technical questions of medical care. It symbolized the larger anxieties of the upper middle classes about the new forms of industrialization, urbanization, and immigration that were quickly changing the face of everyday relations in the United States. Many middle-class citizens who traced their ancestry to Anglo-Protestant origins feared that these new immigrants could not assimilate and would ultimately destroy the fabric of American society. They translated the differences in religion, language, and culture between themselves and these new immigrants into ideas about "whiteness" and consequently the qualities for assimilation. Thus, because the rise in working-class immigration from eastern and southern Europe as well as from Mexico in the late nineteenth century created a new demand for midwives across the nation, city officials, physicians, and reformers alike viewed midwives as "non-white" women whose influence would only prevent acculturation. The reformer's race and class-based anxieties about immigrants were thus directly linked to their efforts to curtail midwifery. Their success in getting Los Angeles to take over the role of the midwife ultimately institutionalized their racial assumptions by limiting the practice of midwifery to marginalized women who were foreign born in particular Japanese and Italian.

The declining birth rate among native-born women and the high rate among foreign-born immigrants led many of the upper and middle classes to worry that their peers were committing a form of "race suicide." The scapegoating of midwives for the alarming rates of infant mortality early in the century linked such racist alarms directly to questions about midwifery and medicine. Statistics lent a sense of urgency to the problem. In the 1880s, the U.S. Bureau of the Census began compiling mortality statistics and, in 1915, added birth registration to its records. At the local level, New York City began investigating infant and maternal mortality rates in the late 1900s. Consequently, a picture began to emerge that many found frightening. In 1910, the national infant mortality rate was 124 deaths per 1,000 live births compared to 106 in Great Britain.[3] Mistakenly, as the historical evidence later showed, midwives were blamed.[4]

During this time, Los Angeles enjoyed a lower infant mortality rate than the national average, a rate lower than that of other major cities. Where New York's was 144 per thousand in 1907, in Los Angeles it was 112.[5] (Eventually these numbers began to even out in the 1920s at approximately 70 per thousand for both New York and Los Angeles.)[6] Additionally, a 1912 national survey showed that midwives attended only 10 percent of all births in Los Angeles.[7] Midwives, however, still came under attack in Los Angeles as they did nationally. Los Angeles outpaced many cities in its rate of growth from 1900 to 1910; its population jumped 212 percent.[8] Accompanying this population growth was an increase of births within Los Angeles from 1,590 in 1900 to 5,783 in 1910, a statistic that did not go unnoticed by health officials.[9] That almost 40 percent of these infants had been born to foreign-born parents contributed to the local prejudice against midwives because immigrants made up the majority of their clientele.

Across the nation, physicians used infant mortality rates as an excuse to attack midwifery with government support. Still, many leading physicians believed that an immediate elimination of midwives was impracticable as well as dangerous. Instead, they thought that current medical trends would eventually make the midwife obsolete. As a result, these medical practitioners called for regulation rather than elimination. They relied on studies from Great Britain that showed that licensing midwives contributed toward lowering infant mortality rates.[10] Consequently, the battle that ensued nationwide focused on eliminating the unlicensed midwife. The story of Los Angeles, in this respect, resembles the stories told throughout the major cities of the United States during this period. Los Angeles, however, appears to have been uniquely successful in realizing this goal.

In the late nineteenth century, physicians in Los Angeles attempted to raise the stature of obstetrics by undermining the practice of midwifery. They tried to influence public opinion through rhetoric and through public policy. Their local trade journal, the *Southern California Practitioner*, provides a means to observe this process. Physicians used the periodical to share medical information on obstetrical techniques, especially the use of forceps and chloroform.[11] In February 1906, there were enough physicians (thirty) working exclusively in obstetrics to form their own subsection within the county medical society.[12] The journal's pages record the ways in which local physicians endeavored to control the birth experience and the limits to their efforts.

In general, physicians contended that midwives lacked a scientific understanding of disease transmission and, thus, constituted a public health danger. In 1895, the *Southern California Practitioner* argued that "physicians practicing in our large cities have learned to associate the midwife and puerperal fever, and regard her as an evil of great magnitude."[13] Local physicians maintained that crafting hygienic hands—the primary means for preventing infection—was not a simple procedure. Instead they considered it an intricate process: washing up to one's elbows, scrub brushing in a sublimate solution for five minutes, using fresh water to rinse, and repeating the entire procedure. The *Southern California Practitioner* argued that "all this takes time, but if by repeating it and taking other antiseptic precautions a thousand times we can prevent one attack of septicemia, it will be well worth our while."[14] The journal implied that physicians were schooled in such methods and midwives were not.

Local physicians recognized the public's favor toward midwives over doctors in attending births: "Often men of true science and ability are obliged to stand aside by popular opinion and view the malpractice of the ignorant midwife."[15] If they wanted to make any inroads, they knew they needed to change public attitudes. They contended that birth needed to be understood as a complicated medical procedure rather than simply an ordinary event. In particular, the editors of the *Southern California Practitioner* argued that the unpredictable character of the childbirth experience made specialized knowledge imperative: "No matter how healthy the woman or how normal the pregnancy, no one can guarantee there may not be a complication in labor which will demand, if not baffle, all the skill that an educated physician can give."[16] When it went wrong, the dangers were catastrophic for women, children, and families. In their discourse, the editors used the word "midwifery" to connote bad practice: "Incompetent practitioners, not all of them on the illegal list either, by their dirty and meddlesome midwifery occasion, and in the minds of some justify such talk."

Yet, despite arguments by physicians to pay deference to the obstetrician, local specialists were scarce. In 1887, the *Southern California Practitioner* hailed the establishment of a gynecological and obstetrical hospital by Walter Lindley and Francis L. Haynes as an advantage for all of the Southwest, including Arizona and New Mexico. While Lindley and Haynes intended their institution to serve for the "Especial Treatment of Gynecological and Lying-In Patients," they initially allowed physicians to apply to use the facility for treating other ailments.[17] Evidently, they needed the extra income.

In addition to printing rhetorical attacks and publicizing the existence of alternate facilities, the *Southern California Practitioner* published eyewitness testimony from chief health officer Luther Milton Powers to call into question the competence of midwives. On October 17, 1890, Catherine E. Smith called Powers at five in the morning to attend a woman who had given birth prematurely by two months.[18] Powers arrived on the scene to find the woman "pale, anxious, almost pulseless, and had other symptoms of severe shock." Between the woman's thighs lay what looked like "a large smooth compressible tumor about the size of her head ... with the placenta and membrane partly attached." Powers concluded that "[he] had an inverted uterus to replace." The placenta had failed to separate from the uterine wall, pulling the uterus outside the woman's body when the placenta exited, creating a life-threatening situation. Why did it invert, he asked? He informed his readers that this condition "occur[ed] very seldom, but more frequently in precipitate labors, instrumental deliveries, in primiparae, those suffering from some nervous disturbance and in the service of midwives and ignorant attendants." In this case Powers decided that "taking into consideration the character of the midwife and the extensive inversion of the vagina, [he was] inclined to think that traction of the cord, and pressure over the abdomen completed the inversion." He took the fact that "the midwife denied everything" as proof of her culpability.

The pages of the *Southern California Practitioner* document the local elite's philosophical and personal challenges to midwifery. Local physicians also attempted to use the municipal board of health to change the city's medical social geography. In 1889, the physician-controlled board of health instructed the health officer to devise an ordinance to register midwives. Cataloging, presumably, created a means for supervision. Yet, after taking this step, the board appears to have taken no action on applications. In fact, the subject of midwives disappears from the minutes until 1899.[19] At that point, the minutes reference a subcommittee on midwifery, whose responsibility was to draft recommendations on applications for permits. Between 1899 and 1904, the board recommended that the city grant five permits and deny eight. Unfortunately, the minutes are moot on the reasons behind the board's decisions.

Despite taking action, these records reveal the board's weak authority in these matters. Further evidence of their powerlessness was evidenced by the fact that the board felt it necessary to pass a motion on August 5, 1902, "order[ing] that no midwives be allowed to register until passed upon by the Board of Health." Apparently midwives could and did bypass the board. In addition, midwives who were denied a permit did not necessarily passively accept the board's decision. In a case briefly publicized in the *Los Angeles Times* in 1904, Louisa Claussen challenged the validity of the city's ordinance regulating midwifery in the local courts.[20] While the newspaper did not report any follow-up, the scant evidence that exists suggests that she reached a stalemate with the city. While Claussen's name never appeared again in the board of health minutes detailing recommendations on permits, she kept advertising her practice in the business section of the city directory.

Three years later, in 1907, the board of health brought their problems to Mayor Harper's attention. They identified language as a major issue in enforcement. Many of the immigrant women who came for an examination did not speak English, making it difficult for the board to assess their professionalism. One board of health member described his encounter with Dominga C. Franco, a Mexican midwife.[21] She arrived at his office with a certificate from a Mexican medical college but, because she spoke only Spanish, he could not actually converse with her. As a result, he did not feel that he could adequately conduct an interview. Still, he supposed that her credential was probably good and that she "knew the art." Whether it was her degree or her demeanor that convinced him of her creditability remains a mystery. Powers also related to the mayor that a lack of public support proved the second major inhibitor. Powers said, "Public sentiment seems to help [the midwives] some." Mayor Harper reacted to this report by commanding the board to renew enforcement attempts and "prosecute fake midwives" for practicing without a license.

In combination, this archival evidence suggest that although the board of health created administrative rules requiring licensure, it was unable to enforce them. Even more suggestive is the fact that although the board identified enforcement as a problem, an analysis of its minutes from 1905 to 1911 indicates that they did not deny a permit to any woman who applied.[22] Moreover, only thirty-five women applied to the board for permits during this period, and once they obtained a license very few registered again. This absence of action can be understood as a quiet admission of the board's lack of power. Thus, it appears that while local elite physicians desired to rid the city of midwives, they were stymied as to how to accomplish that feat.

Perceiving the city's laxity, female reformers felt compelled to take up the battle against the midwife. Maude Foster Weston spearheaded these efforts during her tenure as the superintendent of the Los Angeles College Settlement Association's (LACSA) district nursing program from 1898 to 1913. She guided investigations into the relationship between infant mortality and obstetrical service and concluded that midwives were to blame. Her opinion echoed beliefs of the settlement workers and the medical establishment nationwide. Weston's concern was not solely altruistic. From her perspective, midwives directly competed with public health nurses for medical authority. She felt that the public, especially immigrants, mistakenly viewed midwives as the greater experts on questions related to the health of women and children than her nurses. As a result, Weston viewed midwifery as an impediment to her attempts to establish a unique place for public health nursing within the city's health care hierarchy as well as the public's favor. In response, she devised two different strategies to eliminate the midwife from the medical landscape: reporting and replacement. Ultimately Weston's combination of surveillance with the project of substitution resulted in the broadest interpretation of public health and civic application of services seen so far in the city's history.

Since the district nursing program's inception, Weston had forbidden public health nurses from accepting any case "where a Midwife has been or is in attendance."[23] By denying services, Weston hoped to persuade poor women to abandon what she believed to be archaic remedies in favor of the modern medical techniques offered by the public health nurse. More importantly, her policy excluded recalcitrant women from access to a specialist because, in 1907, Weston had secured municipal funds for a maternity nurse.

By being in charge of the physical environment during the birth and obligated to provide assistance afterwards, the maternity nurse's responsibilities mimicked some of the tasks performed by midwives. At the time of delivery, the maternity nurse created a sanitary setting for the birth, being "responsible for the cleanliness of the patient, her bed and her room." The maternity nurse's responsibilities also included maintaining watch during the lying-in period, the ten days after birth. Weston was determined, however, to set the maternity nurse's work apart from that of midwives. She required the nurse to conduct "as many Ante-partum and Advisory Visits" as she could to instruct the expectant parents about prenatal care. She also lent "needy cases" linen and materials to construct baby clothes.[24]

The sharpest distinction was that the maternity nurse did not deliver babies. Instead, she offered something presumably better in Weston's opinion: modern medical science. Based on this belief, Weston enlisted the help of medical students from the College of Medicine. The *Southern California Practitioner* had floated the idea of using students to attend indigent puerperal cases a few years earlier. Reprinting an editorial from *Obstetrics*, the journal argued it would be mutually beneficial; students would gain clinical experience at the same time that the needs of the poor would be served. The journal suggested that students were better than midwives: "The transportation of obstetrical clinical experience from the midwife to the educatable [sic] student of medicine will prove of greater advantage to all women in confinement than would a specific cure for puerperal infection."[25] Many medical schools did in fact turn this idea into practice in the 1920s.[26] Los Angeles, thus, appears to be a leader in this movement.

Detailed rules dictated the division of responsibility between medical students and maternity nurses. Weston explicitly forbade the nurses from conducting internal examinations unless an emergency arose. She also stipulated that the students, not the nurse, ensure that the infant's eyes receive a drop of silver nitrate to prevent blindness from venereal disease. Yet, the student's authority was not without limits. Medical students could not perform operations without the presence of the supervising obstetrician. In terms of personal conduct, Weston warned the nurses not to "criticize the treatment order nor question the methods employed by the students." Reciprocally, the rules instructed medical students to "act in a courteous manner towards the patient and the nurse."[27] In theory, these codes muted confrontations in front of patients. They also established a mutually dependent, albeit hierarchical relationship between nurses and physicians.

While the rules applied to all the nurses working in the program, they were particularly important for the one nurse whom Weston had designated to work exclusively with maternity patients. We know very little about Cordelia E. Macy, the program's maternity nurse from 1908 to 1913. What little we can glean from the 1920 and 1930 U.S. Census manuscripts and the program's reports is that she was an experienced nurse in her early thirties, that she had graduated from the Mary Hitchcock Memorial Hospital in Hanover, New Hampshire, and that she had worked in the Manhattan Hospital of New York. From her reports we know that she was busy.

Macy's predecessor treated 182 patients from 1907 to 1908.[28] Macy attended slightly more than double that number in her first year and approximately four hundred patients each year after that. Although Macy's records indicate that her patients were ethnically diverse, they would have all been considered "non-white" by white, middle-class women's standards. Mexicans composed the largest percentage of Macy's patients, rising from 64 percent to

83 percent from 1910 to 1913. These numbers reflect residential segregation as well as the influx of Mexicans migrating to Los Angeles to escape the turmoil of the Mexican Revolution. The next largest groups, Italians and Russian Jews, each formed 5 percent to 6 percent of Macy's clientele. Very few of Macy's cases were unmarried, deserted by their husbands, or widows. Nor did it appear that they were destitute. Their husbands' average wages amounted to $1.50 a day, which was just slightly under the average advertised in the newspapers for general laborers.[29] Thus, the majority of the program's clientele had the resources to pursue a variety of medical therapies, although private hospitalization was probably outside of their means.

The stories told in the chapter on public health nursing detail the ambivalent relationship of immigrants toward the efforts of female reformers. Based on these records it appears that women and their families accessed the settlement's program before, during, and after childbirth. The nurse's records also indicate that patients discriminated among the instructions they were given to follow. Whether the visits were initiated by the nurse or by patients and their families, the sheer number Macy rendered made her a significant source of medical care.

Even though Macy attended to patients in all nine wards, the Eighth Ward always comprised her largest percentage. One visitor from the East Coast who was interested in LACSA's work commented, "Oh, this is more like it," as he toured the Eighth Ward and confronted "eastern standards of poverty, wretchedness and congestion of habitation."[30] A sense of familiarity was perhaps provoked even further by the presence of "a goodly number of Jews." Throughout the program's annual reports, Weston commonly conflated "non-white" immigrants and their dwellings with disease. For instance, she described how the Second Ward had slowly evolved into an area of substandard housing, where the "Mexican adobe and patio ... have become ill-smelling, tuberculosis-breeding tenements." Even when she did not describe any squalor, Weston believed that the mere presence of Mexicans, Italians, and African Americans made their neighborhoods prime candidates for public health. The settlement's work in housing reform reinforced her assumptions.

Weston found the environmental conditions of these wards particularly troubling for childbearing. In an average year, thousands of women gave birth in the city of Los Angeles. In 1911, the health department recorded 5,792 births, of which 122 were stillbirths and 99 premature infants who subsequently died.[31] In addition, the health officer calculated that another 375 children under the age of one died from diseases of "early infancy" in that same year. At an address before the Conference of Social Workers in Los Angeles in May 1912, Weston said,

"If I could depict in vivid colors the wretched surroundings of most of the mothers and babies who come under the care of our maternity nurse, I know it would not only arouse your sympathy but your indignation."[32] She noted that "besides the eight beds at the County Hospital, and the eleven beds at the maternity Cottage on Utah street, there is no place where that precious charge—the expectant mother—can find care, rest, and refreshment while she awaits the coming of the future citizen of this city." The lack of a maternity hospital reinforced Weston's disdain for midwifery because midwife-attended births took place within the home.

Weston was not alone in her concerns. In 1907, the same year that she secured funding for a maternity nurse, other middle-class white women in Los Angeles established institutions devoted to delivery services. Elizabeth Baurhyte founded the Women's Alliance Maternity Cottage and another group refinanced the Florence Crittenton Home.[33] Marital status dictated assistance. The Crittenton Home aided "unfortunate girls in their most tragic hour," while the Maternity Cottage provided "care of needy wives."[34] The Maternity Cottage prided itself on providing physicians rather than students to attend patients. It also possessed the only baby incubator in the city. These services were not free, however, and in 1920 Baurhyte estimated the charge at twenty-five to thirty-five dollars per patient, an amount in accordance with standard obstetrical fees but too expensive for many immigrant working-class women.[35] In contrast, midwife fees tended to be considerably less.[36] Baurhyte calculated that 203 women used her service from July 1, 1914, to July 1, 1915. In comparison only seventy women used the Crittenton Home during that same period. Although the Maternity Cottage continued to exist throughout the 1920s, the number of women using the facility had dropped to eighty in 1919 even though the capacity had increased from eleven to eighteen.[37]

During the 1890s and early 1900s, only a limited number of other facilities existed for birthing outside the home that might have spawned competition for midwives. In 1900, the Mitchell's Obstetric Hospital and the Woman's Hospital advertised in the city directory but did not appear there in later years. A few more institutions ran listings in the late 1900s: St. Anne's Maternity Hospital, a second Woman's Hospital, and a Women's Sanitary Maternity Home. These hospitals, however, only advertised for one or two years and then disappeared. In addition to these, the Salvation Army Rescue and Maternity Home provided services for a small number of patients throughout the 1900s and 1910s. Typically, these were unmarried women, and the Salvation Army often tried to return them to their families before they gave birth.

Thus, outside the Los Angeles College Settlement's program there existed few charitable or commercial alternatives to midwifery. Obstetricians were scarce and expensive. Maternity hospitals were few. The combination led Weston to complain in 1912 that the "struggle with the midwife is ceaseless. A number of them are in the city. Some have been here for years."[38] While she had always prohibited the public health nurses from working in conjunction with a midwife, in 1910 she further ordered the nurses to report names and addresses of unlicensed midwives they encountered to the city health office. While Weston found encouragement from the establishment of alternative facilities, she looked toward the city to take a more active role in protecting infant and maternal health. She created services, but she desired the city to act on its ordinances and enforce its regulations.

Public health officials could only regulate what they could see. As a result, Weston's and the city's efforts to control the practice of midwifery in Los Angeles concentrated not on the elusive and traditional practice of female relatives and neighbors but on those women who advertised their wares. Historically, midwifery had been an important means by which women could provide for their family's financial stability.[39] During the late nineteenth century, a number of women established commercial practices in Los Angeles. Undoubtedly, Weston was referring to these women in her complaints. Clearly, not all midwives advertised, but combining this material with census records provides a picture about some of the women who did.[40] Judging by the city directories, over hundred midwives practiced in Los Angeles from 1888 to 1932. Based on these records, approximately 75 percent of these midwives were from Europe (43 percent of whom were German) and 25 percent were from Mexico and Japan.[41]

During the 1890s and 1900s, Mary Spiker, Augusta Bundy, Anna Mueller, Louisa Claussen, Emma Bergstedt, and Wiebcke Kruse consistently advertised in the business section of the city directory. Each of these women practiced anywhere from sixteen to thirty nine years. Census manuscripts indicate that these midwives were more often foreign born than the general population of Los Angeles, a fact that contributed to the association of midwives as "nonwhite" women. Some of these midwives were widowed, some divorced, some married. In general, their labor served as an important, if not primary, source of support for their families. The listings in the city directory suggest that in married households, these women's occupations remained the same throughout this period of time while their husbands and sons changed jobs with greater frequency. Most of these women lived within immigrant neighborhoods just south of downtown. Even as the city began to annex towns to the northwest, south, and southwest during the 1890s, the midwives residences' stayed relatively stable. Two women, Bundy and Mueller, eventually acquired property slightly farther out of downtown during the first decade of the twentieth century, perhaps mirroring the movements of some of their clientele.

If the city directories are correct, Anna Mueller practiced midwifery longer than any of the others. Born in Germany in 1841, Mueller registered with the California State Board of Health until she was ninety one. Married to Michael Mueller, a saloon keeper, Anna Mueller continued working long after her husband retired. From 1899 to 1900, the Muellers shared a rented home at 519 East First Street with their son-in-law, daughter, and infant granddaughter—Joseph, Lena, and Violet Warder. The Muellers also probably supported the extended family because Joseph worked only sporadically as a waiter. Thanks in no small part to Anna's practice, which included many Chinese patients, the Muellers owned 1218 Maple Avenue free of mortgage by 1920. Mueller also found favor with the board of health, which always recommended she be granted a permit.[42]

Augusta Bundy was born in Norway the same year as Mueller. She maintained her listing in the city directory from 1888 to 1915, when she would have been seventy three years old. Bundy was married but did not have any children. She and her husband, Arthur T. Bundy, moved several times during their early years in Los Angeles, perhaps to be near Arthur's various jobs. He tried mining gold, working as a cement worker, and owning his own shop, Bundy & Sears, which sold wood, coal, hay, and grain. Not until 1898 did he achieve some stability as the foreman for the Paraffine Paint Company, a job he held for the next several years. Combined with Augusta's regular practice as a midwife, this allowed the couple, now in the their sixties, to buy a home at 2093 Miranda Street. The timing was fortunate. Within months, the now elderly Arthur was taking whatever odd jobs he could find.[43]

Mary Spiker was born in Germany, a year before Mueller and Bundy. By 1900 she had lived in California for at least thirty years. Unlike Mueller and Bundy, Spiker was divorced. She owned her own home on Hewitt Street in which she kept a boardinghouse to supplement her income as a midwife. Over the course of her life she had given birth to ten children, six of whom were still alive in 1900, three of whom she directly supported. Her two sons started off employed as blacksmiths and tobacconists, but over the years they took less skilled jobs as common laborers and roofers. Consequently, Spiker's work as a boardinghouse keeper and midwife maintained her family.[44]

Without census data, Louisa Claussen, Wiebcke Kruse, and Emma Bergstedt's lives are harder to decipher. Their last names indicate that they were probably of German descent. All three were widows. Kruse helped support two men, most likely her children, who lived in her household until 1902. One worked as a carpet weaver while the other worked as a bookbinder. Claussen's household included two men who were probably her sons. At first Henry Claussen tried to make a living as a musician but became a fireman and later an engineer for the Santa Fe Railroad because, presumably, these positions paid more and provided greater job security. Herman Claussen worked as a boiler maker but later became a bartender. Bergstedt lived alone and eventually moved to what is now South Pasadena. The stability of Claussen, Kruse, and Bergstedt's work can be partially judged by the fact that they lived at a single residence for the majority of the time that they advertised their practices.[45]

Thus, a number of women had active midwifery practices in Los Angeles at the turn of the twentieth century. While certainly more women practiced than are discussed here, detailing even the basic outlines of their lives gives a sense of the viability of their practices and puts a face to a forgotten history. In the 1910s, their place within the city's health care system changed.

In 1910, when Maude Foster Weston's success at supplanting the midwives with a maternity nurse was still uncertain and the city's initial endeavors at legislation had proven to be weak, the arrest and conviction of Catherine E. Smith added new strength to the movement against the midwife. Smith, a native of West Virginia, founded Bellevue Lying-in Hospital in 1887 primarily to serve as an unofficial adoption center.[46] She described her institution as a place "where children, fatherless or motherless, receive care, comfort and attention and find a good home."[47] By 1894, she claimed that she had taken care of five hundred cases. Smith's success, however, also made her an object of closer scrutiny, and her actions in a famous kidnapping case led to more stringent regulation of midwifery in the city.

The first issue that made Smith suspect, and other midwives so by association, was her claim on medical knowledge. She advertised in the city directory as "Mrs. Dr. J. H. Smith" although she had never obtained a license from an accredited medical college. Consequently, the state board of medical examiners identified her as an "illegal" practitioner and pressured her to desist her false advertising. Smith acquiesced for a brief period of time but in 1901 she again placed "Dr." back into her advertisements and stated her occupation in the census as "Doctress." At the municipal level, Smith had first become suspect to city officials in the 1890s when Powers implicated her in writing about obstetrical cases.[48] The city board of health denied Smith a permit to maintain her lying-in hospital in 1908, and while she made appeals they continued to refuse her request through the next year.[49]

The trial of Catherine Smith in 1910 proved a sensation in Los Angeles; however, the exact charge was baby stealing, not midwifery. The case began in January 1910, when a Mrs. Wilson, wife of a druggist, reportedly gave birth to a set of quadruplets. What seemed so unbelievable was that Wilson had previously given birth to two sets of triplets for which, reportedly, President

Theodore Roosevelt had sent her an autographed picture with a letter of congratulation.[50] (Roosevelt's interest reflected a common belief among the upper-middle classes that intelligence and moral character were inherited traits and that, consequently, "white" women should propagate to ensure the future of America's greatness as a nation.) The *Los Angeles Daily Examiner* reported that large numbers of women descended upon the Wilson house in the hopes of seeing the four babies, only to be turned away, and the next day the paper quickly exposed that it was a hoax.[51]

On January 25, 1910, three days after the initial report of the births, Catherine Smith entered the picture. Smith had brokered the unofficial adoption. Her daughter, Lena Hayes, had pretended to act as Wilson's nurse but, in fact, had sneaked the unrelated babies into Wilson's house from elsewhere. With scandal brewing, Smith paid a visit to Wilson. Smith demanded that Wilson return the infants so that she could give them back to their original parents, but "after an altercation with Mrs. Wilson, Mrs. Smith retired without the babies." In speaking with the police, Smith had originally stated that she had secured the four babies from the county hospital, from the Clara Barton Hospital, and from a saleswoman and a physician. Smith also told reporters that she had placed over three hundred children in new homes and that "her secrets . . . if revealed, would create a sensation."[52]

Since 1908, the health department had denied Smith a permit for running a lying-in hospital. Consequently, she steadfastly stuck by her story that none of the babies had been born in her institution. When Wilson appeared in court, she contended that she was motivated by "mother love" and she turned on Smith. Wilson stated that Smith had "inveighed her into the scheme," and that Smith typically received monetary compensation from interested parties who wanted to rid themselves of a child. By doing so, Wilson portrayed Smith as being devoid of proper feminine feelings or manners. She played to gender assumptions that might forgive certain transgressions if they were thought to stem from a woman's biological nature and, in turn, helped criminalize midwives whose commercial practices might be portrayed as an affront to womanly behavior. It was also at this point in the story that it became apparent that one of the infants had been born at the Smith residence. Smith risked prosecution and explained that this was a "charity case" who had duped Smith by using a false name and subsequently disappeared. She declared that she did not know the true identity of the mother. Soon thereafter, Sadie Engleman came forward and brought a civil suit against Smith for kidnapping her baby, asking the court for $5,000.

As for Wilson, her "mother love" won out in the end. In June, at the same time as the conclusion of the Smith trial, the court granted Wilson custody of the older children who had been a part of the previous triplet hoaxes. As for the "quadruplets," Engleman's child had died in the city's custody while another baby had been returned to its birth mother and, after winning her case, Wilson put in an application to obtain custody of the other two infants.[53]

Smith found herself in court five months after the scandal broke. Technically the charge was for stealing Engleman's child; however, her status as a midwife was used as a means to question her character. Engleman alleged a tale of lost innocence. At the age of sixteen, Engleman moved to San Diego from Los Angeles. After working in laundries for a bit, she became a chorus girl and changed her name to Bessie Wise. Falling in love with a sailor, who supposedly made promises of marriage, Engleman engaged in intimate relations. She returned to Los Angeles once she found herself pregnant. She accused Smith of taking the baby the day after its birth. In Smith's version, Engleman's mother begged Smith to take in the girl but Smith refused. She advised her to seek help at the county hospital, but the girl showed up at her doorstep anyway. After the birth, according to Smith, Engleman took little interest in her own child.

The newspapers meticulously recorded Smith's courtroom demeanor. During the first days of the trial, Smith reportedly "took great interest in the proceedings and indicated her disagreement with much of the evidence by a vigorous shaking of her head at certain stages of the narrative." During her own testimony, "the old lady beamed benevolently upon the jury, and when she talked she looked straight into the face of every man on the panel." Could Smith convince them of her maternal nature? Although allegedly fifty-five, the newspapers believed Smith to be much older: she was sixty. After five hours of deliberations, Smith seemed unfazed as the jury read the verdict of guilty on the charge of child stealing. According to the *Times*, "When the verdict was read, the stoicism of the Sioux Indian as he gladly goes to his death hoping to meet the great Father on the Happy Hunting Grounds was typified in the face of the woman. Women friends around her wept copiously, but she gave no sign." During the sentencing phase, Smith apparently began to appear fatigued to the point of collapse, which the *Times* attributed to her recognition of her plight.[54]

The connection between Smith's actions in the Engleman case, the quadruplet scandal, and her work as a midwife became apparent upon conviction. According to the *Los Angeles Times*, "The convicted woman has been in the midwife profession in this city many years. She has been mixed in unsavory transactions. But this is the first time she has been caught." Part of her claim for leniency in sentencing and appeal for probation hinged on her willingness to cease practicing midwifery and to allow the Southern California Medical Association to maintain surveillance of her actions to ensure compliance.

Smith's probation officer appealed for a character reference from the board of health. Upon his request, the board met in special session on June 28, 1910, to discuss whether it should lend its support for leniency. The *Times* printed a transcript of the impassioned discussion.

> "This woman has defied the health department for years," said [Health Officer Powers], "and it is fortunate that she has been tried before a court and a judge that would convict her."
>
> "I know the woman myself," said the Mayor [Alexander], "and I think she ought to be put out of business. She is no different from any other criminal and she has denied the authorities for years."
>
> "Still," said Dr. Clark, "the attitude of this board may send her to prison. I would not want to vote with that as a result."
>
> "Well, I would," said Dr. [George L.] Cole. "I will do it right now. Years ago I told this woman to stop her nefarious work and told her that I would aid in sending her to prison if I could. I am ashamed that a few physicians defended her because—well, because there was good reason to do so, but I feel that her punishment is well deserved."
>
> Prof. Stabler asked what the Board of Health had to do with the case anyway. "Nothing," said Dr. Cole, who moved that the board do nothing that would impede sentence on the woman to the penitentiary. The mayor put the motion and it was passed unanimously.[55]

While the board believed Smith to be innocent on the charge of baby stealing, they refused to help her based on their past disagreements. Their opposition to probation focused on her history as a midwife, not the singular evidence presented in the Engleman case. Nonetheless, the probation officer persuaded Judge Davis to free Smith from jail on the condition that she stop practicing midwifery and permanently sever any connections to maternity homes or lying-in hospitals. While satisfactory to the probation officer, Smith "grumbled audibly against [the stipulations] as she left the courtroom."[56]

The Smith trial proved pivotal in changing the attitudes of city officials toward midwives. The courtroom drama, which the city's major newspapers widely publicized, undoubtedly facilitated an association between baby brokering, unhealthy delivery practices, and midwifery. Its resolution also suggested that legal action could be an effective strategy for curtailment. Weston seized the moment to argue that without a vigorous law the nurses could "only hope for partial success" in reigning in the offending practitioners.[57] Three weeks after the Smith trial's conclusion, on July 19, 1910, the city council approved a new ordinance to regulate midwifery in Los Angeles.

Unlike the board's previous attempts, Ordinance 20,606 made it illegal for a person to engage in midwifery without first obtaining a permit. They based the criteria, however, not on having a diploma from an accredited school but, instead, on experience and moral character. This reflected practical realities because very few midwifery schools existed within the United States. Moreover, the general public was just beginning to view birth as an event needing specialized knowledge that could not be learned solely through experience. The city would not grant a permit if the board of health determined that the applicant had engaged in an immoral or criminal act. The permits were good for one year, and could be renewed for a dollar. Persons who did not comply were guilty of a misdemeanor and subject to a fine ranging from five to five hundred dollars and jail time no longer than six months.

In spite of the passage of the 1910 ordinance that limited the practice of midwives, public health reformers remained dissatisfied with the public's reliance on midwifery. In 1914, midwives admitted to having attended to at least 1,082 (14 percent) of the total 7,757 births in Los Angeles.[58] While this percentage was not very great compared to national estimates, the overall growth of the population of Los Angeles along with a rapidly rising birth rate during the 1910s prompted their concern. In 1910, the U.S. Bureau of the Census estimated that Los Angeles had a population a little over 100,000, and by 1920 this figured had tripled. At the same time, the city health department estimated that the number of births had almost doubled, from approximately 5,800 to 10,800 in 1920. Although the department did not break these numbers down by race or ethnicity, the steady rise in numbers of southern and eastern Europeans might have provoked a concern not only about the rising birth rate but, more importantly, about who was giving birth.[59]

Questions of medical authority overlapped with issues of immigration. In retrospect, the head of the division, Lyle G. McNeile, argued that prior to the formation of the municipal program expectant mothers were at risk for two reasons.[60] On the one hand, he believed that "Los Angeles with its large foreign population, many of whom are indigent, was largely dependent upon midwives." Second, he asserted that LACSA's use of "medical students who acted without supervision, for the care of a large number of women during pregnancy, labor and the lying-in period" was problematic.

Given the limited institutional options, the health department built upon Weston's original initiatives. Formed in September 1915, the Division of Obstetrics (renamed in 1920 as the Maternity Division) was headed by physician Lyle G. McNeile and run by his wife, physician Olga McNeile.[61] The creation of this division culminated the various attempts to eliminate midwifery from the medical landscape of Los Angeles. Weston and public health officials' frustrations with regulation would be resolved if the division made midwifery obsolete. As reiterated by the *Los Angeles Times*, "efficient medical service ... eliminates the undesirable midwife."[62] Printing notices in English, Spanish, Italian, French, and Slavonian, the city publicized the formation of the service to its various immigrant communities. Importantly, it emphasized the availability of free home care.

After touring facilities nationwide, McNeile boasted that Los Angeles's program was the "first and largest municipal maternity service in the world."[63] He argued that although prenatal care had become standard practice in health departments throughout the United States, "the establishment of a [municipal] dispensary which would actually supervise the care of the prospective mother throughout pregnancy, would care for her at the time of delivery, and would provide medical and nursing supervision during the lying-in period, was an innovation." By providing for a home birth and assistance afterwards, the division directly competed with the midwife. In order to fulfill its duties, the Division of Obstetrics was a private-public joint venture, or as the *Los Angeles Times* dubbed it in 1914, "semi-municipal." The city maintained administrative power but utilized private personnel and facilities to carry out its work. The service cost the city a little less than five dollars per application in 1917 and had increased to only eight dollars by 1923.[64]

The Neighborhood House Settlement provided space for a central headquarters at 1320 Wilson Street, which McNeile described as being "in the heart of the congested district," a euphemism for an immigrant neighborhood. The settlement remodeled these facilities within the first year to include a sleeping porch, office, living room, shower, bath, and toilet. These arrangements allowed two senior medical students from the College of Physicians and Surgeons, Medical Department, University of Southern California, to work for two weeks straight. These students did not handle actual labor calls alone. McNeile required the presence of a licensed physician for supervision, and he was able to convince a number of local physicians to volunteer their time. The Los Angeles County Medical Association also donated its telephone exchange for the city's service. By mandating that the staff members call in every forty-five minutes, McNeile felt that prompt attendance would be ensured. A new system in 1920 allowed the division to reach any physician within fifteen minutes.

Despite technological advances that might have changed perceptions of urban space, McNeile still expressed concerns related to the rapid territorial growth of the city. Patients and practitioners ceased to be neighbors, and this separation raised a number of different problems, many of which were financial. At the time of the division's establishment in 1915, the city had just extended its borders from 107.62 square miles to 284.89. Five years later, Los Angeles annexed another seventeen towns and extended its territory another 80 square miles.[65] Getting around the city cost money. Students and volunteer physicians paid for their own carfare, which McNeile estimated at two-and-a half to twelve dollars each week. Theoretically the expansion of new technologies of communication should have allowed for more efficient interaction between patient and physician, but the expense of phone calls limited its usefulness. McNeile noted that he had "received many reports showing that our patients were unable to call us, and were delivered without attendance because on account of their destitute circumstances they did not possess the necessary five cents."[66] Despite his reservations, McNeile emphasized the importance of the telephone even more as the city continued to grow geographically.

The Division of Obstetrics used the health department's central headquarters as an administrative office. The division ran two maternity dispensaries in separate locations to provide prenatal care. Again, local settlement houses provided the facilities. The Neighborhood House Settlement donated space for one dispensary around the corner from its central headquarters. The Brownson Settlement, which was located in a Russian, Greek, Mexican, Italian, and French community, provided the other. Each dispensary was open for half a day each week, and McNeile put his wife, physician Olga McNeile, in charge. Olga McNeile ran the dispensaries until she and her husband separated, and later divorced in 1920. In 1918, Lyle McNeile argued that having a woman run the dispensaries showed a consideration for the patients, especially in his opinion for the "foreign women . . . who would not otherwise avail themselves of this service." McNeile believed that femininity transcended racial or ethnic differences. For the very same reason, he only employed female clerks. Yet, Olga McNeile was the one female physician hired on a full-time basis until the appointment of Ruth Janetta Temple, an African American physician, in 1924. Fifty-four years later, Temple described McNeile's hesitance in hiring a female obstetrician. Expressing another common turn-of-the-twentieth-century belief about femininity, McNeile considered the schedule too demanding for them.[67]

In order to provide all the amenities of the midwife, particularly during the ten days following the birth, the division turned to the city's nurses. The health department's two-year-old Bureau of Nursing (formerly the Los Angeles College Settlement Association's District Nursing Program coordinated by Maude Foster Weston) supplied the personnel. McNeile found these nurses to be instrumental for patient communication. He noted, "Individual nurses have been of great assistance, not only in their professional work, but in explaining to patients, ignorant and greatly frightened, about the objects of the service, what is to be done and what the result would be."[68] McNeile further remarked that this was crucial for cases that demanded hospitalization but where patients "as a result of ignorance of our customs, would not consent to go."

The nurses became increasingly responsible for policing the service and conducting checks on patients' financial backgrounds. This followed a pattern established by Weston, who in 1910 required the nurses of the LACSA program to report any unlicensed midwives they encountered. Two years later, the city's limited nursing personnel began using its police powers against midwives for failing to register births. The health department's "Special Nurse," Margaret Sirch, commented that a recent conviction against a midwife for this offense had produced a favorable affect in terms of this specific requirement. She also noted that Russian women tended to be guilty of this crime. In order to induce midwives to comply with filing a birth registration, the health department stipulated in 1916 that as a condition of license all midwives had to fill out a birth certificate in English. The nursing administration believed that for registering births "this ruling ha[d] been of inestimable value, as many of the midwives are of foreign birth."[69] By forcing these "non-white" women to use the dominant language, the city hoped they might foster assimilation or force midwives to give up their practice. Despite the officials' desire to use nurses for these various tasks, McNeile worried over problems of authority because the nurses did not work directly under the Division of Obstetrics. McNeile stated that physicians "cannot be expected to reverse the usual order of their professional life, and receive their orders from the nursing division, rather than from a physician whose training has been equal to their own."[70]

The original purpose of the obstetrics division was to provide prenatal care, home delivery, and postnatal care to the "poorer classes" of Los Angeles. McNeile expected women to report to the nearest dispensary at least every two weeks during their pregnancy.[71] There they would receive instruction on the "hygiene of pregnancy" as well as a physical examination including a pelvic exam and urinalysis. Reflecting the needs of its immigrant population, the division printed leaflets in English, German, and Spanish entitled "Advice to Prospective Mothers." McNeile hoped that this information would produce a "material effect upon infant mortality." He ordered physicians on his staff to make house calls when their patients did not report to the dispensary. According to his records, the division made 1,020 prenatal house calls in its first ten months of its existence, approximately twenty-five per week. He also recorded 763 dispensary visits. Considering that there were only two students and that the division only attended 263 women, McNeile might have inflated these numbers. More importantly, these numbers suggest that some women chose to avail themselves of only certain aspects of the program. They might have attended a dispensary once but decided against returning. Or, they might have used the dispensary but decided to use a midwife to birth their childen. Throughout the 1920s, McNeile continued to record enormous numbers of cases visiting the dispensaries relative to the number of deliveries. In 1925, he calculated that the department had delivered 7,285 children, made 27,800 house calls, and conducted 52,322 dispensary visits in its ten years of existence. Two years after the city established the division, McNeile viewed its growth as "conclusive" proof that the division filled a need within the city.

Employees had a different take on the increased workload. In a letter to McNeile dated November 10, 1924, the interns (six at this point) objected to their working conditions for themselves and for their patients: "This is to notify you that conditions in the City Maternity Service are in a chaotic state, and that unless some immediate steps are taken to rectify them, nothing but disaster awaits."[72] Between their work at the dispensary, attending labors, postpartum visits, and responding to "false alarms," they found themselves working twenty-four hours a day. They announced to their supervisor that "physically we are totally depleteded [sic] and our physical unfitness is beginning to tell on the work." They recounted several cases where fatigue led them to make minor mistakes that luckily had not caused greater misfortune. McNeile provided this letter to the city council in asking to expand the program's personnel, requests he repeatedly made throughout the 1920s.[73]

The original purpose of the division was to provide care for women who could not afford a private physician. McNeile assumed that these women would want home deliveries. During the first year, however, he claimed that there had been "an overwhelming demand from pregnant women who wish to be confined at the County Hospital and other allied institutions."[74] By opening the service to women who wanted to go to the hospital rather than being delivered by the service the city could still provide prenatal and postnatal care. Although McNeile perceived this as a pressing demand in 1917, the city still attended almost 90 percent of its patients in their homes.

While the city engaged in a project of substitution, the state of California took measures to eliminate the unlicensed midwife. Following a national trend, in March 1917 the state amended an existing act that regulated the practice of medicine to include midwives. This added midwives to a list that already included physicians, surgeons, and chiropractics who needed to obtain a certificate to practice. The midwife's certificate, however, only allowed her to attend childbirth under normal circumstances. The act required midwives to prove good moral character and show that they had received a diploma from an approved school. The state also stipulated that midwives attend a year-long course from a hospital that would instruct them in anatomy, physiology, obstetrics, hygiene, and sanitation. In addition, midwives needed to pass a state board exam on those subjects. Administered in English, a portion of the exam consisted of a writing section. Taken as a whole, these requirements were difficult to fulfill in the United States and proved prohibitive for many immigrants.[75]

The act did contain one loophole. In deference to practical realities, midwives who had already practiced in California for at least a year prior to the act's passage could apply for a certificate without being subject to the new requirements. These women needed to prove that they attended at least twenty-five cases in the past year to be considered practicing and that they had not only assisted the birth but attended to the woman for ten days after the birth, the "lying-in" period. Furthermore, these women had to prove their "good moral character" by providing two affidavits: one from a physician and the other from a layman, preferably a religious leader.

Although the state mandated a harsher punishment for practicing without a license than that of the city, the chief health officer of Los Angeles, L. M. Powers, expressed reservations. The new state law effectively annulled the city's ordinance, and Powers believed, consequently that this new law jeopardized the city's control. Powers contended that the nullification of the city's laws left it without its own recourse. In response, he proposed a much more restrictive ordinance, which would detail when a midwife could or could not attend a birth. Powers also wanted to mandate exactly what equipment midwives needed to possess and to forbid anything not expressly listed. The city attorney rejected Powers's proposal on legal grounds but, to calm his fears, suggested the city require midwives to register with the city health department in the same manner that physicians, surgeons, and dentists did. In the end, the department refused to register anyone who could not meet the state standards. Even though this law was redundant, it was symbolic.[76]

At the same time that the city's division of obstetrics attempted to replace the midwife, it also served a central function in the new, more overt, attempts by health officials to control the practice. Commensurate with the state legislation, Powers asked the division to conduct investigations of the city's midwives. In his annual report in June 1917, McNeile estimated that "considerable time" had been spent in these endeavors and believed that the new law would in fact "greatly aid this department in enforcing midwife regulations." Under McNeile's direction, the division detected a number of violations and attempted to bring them to court. Yet McNeile also felt that unless the city allocated the funds for him to hire extra nurses to conduct further inspections, he could not follow up on the numerous reports of infractions he was allegedly constantly receiving.[77]

The city prosecuted midwives who did not comply. The city portrayed these women as intractable but, judging by the testimony of one Mexican midwife, confusion rather than resistance led to their noncompliance.[78] According to this midwife's application for state certification, she had lived and practiced midwifery in the United States for forty years. Born in Mexico, during her twenties she had moved to El Paso, Texas, and then relocated with her family to Los Angeles in the 1900s. She was married, had twenty-three children, and did not speak English. According to this midwife's application, she had attended over 1,100 cases and never lost a mother or child. She stated that the board of health in Los Angeles had always granted her a certificate and that her license was current. Consequently, she expressed surprise when she was arrested in late 1919 for practicing without a state license. Considering that the city board had certified her, this midwife did not realize that she was violating any law. She received a suspended sentence of one hundred days in the city jail and was temporarily forbidden from working while she appealed her case to the state board of health. Perhaps because she did not provide an affidavit of births, perhaps because she did not present a school certificate, perhaps because she had never been naturalized, or perhaps because of all or some of these reasons, the state board of health denied this midwife's application for license.

The year after this incident, McNeile believed that the number of investigations that the division had to conduct had "materially decreased" and that those midwives who were working performed with higher quality. McNeile recorded twelve investigations in 1917, twenty in the next year, seventeen in 1919, and then only six in 1920.[79] Los Angeles, it seemed, had eliminated the unlicensed midwife. The city and state's actions, however, opened a space for the practice of midwifery to continue in limited circumstances.

While different in some respects, in its most significant aspect midwifery remained the same in the 1920s as it did at the turn of the twentieth century. It still provided women with a means to financially support their families. Women appealed to the State Board of Medical Examiners to expedite the licensure process because of this burden. One Russian midwife wrote how her husband had been out of work and ill, leaving her to support their four children. She told the board how dire their situation had become, because they had lost all of their possessions and had barely enough to eat. Similarly, a Romanian midwife demanded an urgent answer because she was the sole breadwinner for her mother and daughter.[80]

In addition to their appeals, these women's applications for licenses provide evidence of a number of other similarities between midwifery during the turn of the century and the 1920s. In particular, midwives offered immigrants familiar and affordable health care. The overwhelming majority of midwives in Los Angeles were still foreign born, although their countries of origin had shifted from Europe to Asia. Midwifery in Los Angeles during the 1920s became a Japanese-dominated profession. As early as 1915, one of the city's nurses had noted that the largest number of midwife-supervised births were Japanese.[81] During the 1920s approximately 70 percent of the midwives in Los Angeles listed in the *State Directory of Physicians and Surgeons, Osteopaths, Drugless Practitioners, Chiropodists, and Midwives* were of Japanese heritage. These numbers corresponded to the tremendous growth of Japanese living in Los Angeles after 1910. Many chose to migrate to Los Angeles because of the controversy over segregation in schools in San Francisco and the subsequent Gentleman's Agreement in 1907. In 1900, only 150 Japanese were living in Los Angeles, but by 1920 there were over 10,000 and by 1930 approximately 35,000.[82] This historical coincidence served to reinforce the perception that midwifery was a "non-white" practice.

The general profile of Japanese midwives differed from turn-of-the century European midwives in two ways. First, almost all of the Japanese midwives had graduated from a midwifery school prior to emigrating. In 1877, the Japanese government founded a school for midwives in Tokyo, and a number of private schools were subsequently established in the country's other large cities.[83] These diplomas enabled these women to work within the city, at the same time that the lack of such a credential now increasingly excluded an older generation. Second, judging by their applications, the majority of Japanese midwives were married, but 61 percent did not have children.

In general, the applications to the state suggest that midwives in the 1920s serviced distinct minority populations with whom they shared a common language and culture. The city did not attempt to replicate this aspect in developing its program, which raises one explanation for the limits of its success. In accordance with the 1917 state law, some women submitted affidavits that they had attended twenty-five births. While only a few of these documents exist, they suggest some overall trends. Judging by these documents, Greek midwives attended Greek patients, Italian midwives attended Italian patients, and Japanese midwives attended Japanese patients. The most complete set of affidavits was attached to women's initial applications in 1917. Six women recorded attending a combined total of 113 births in the city of Los Angeles in 1917. Two of these women were Italian, one was French, and three were

Japanese. A few more details about their practices can be gleaned from these documents.

The French midwife worked the least out of the six. She was in her mid-fifties, had children, could speak and read English, and had been living in the United States since the 1890s. She had migrated from France to the state of New York and from there to San Francisco in the early 1900s. The San Francisco earthquake, however, prompted her to move to Los Angeles. Her clientele seemed to be both of French and German origin. During 1917, this midwife attended to only five women, and in the preceding years she recorded a steady but equally small number of cases. Perhaps her age or the small size of the French population in Los Angeles accounts for her relatively light workload. Still, her application indicates that she was not ready to retire.

Unlike this French woman, the two Italian midwives who submitted affidavits had booming businesses that reflected a burgeoning Italian population in the city.[84] Similar to the majority of Japanese applicants, both had obtained university training prior to their arrival in America.[85] They attested to being able to speak and read English only "a little" and all of the names they listed in their written declarations were Italian. These two midwives were almost the same age, one was thirty-eight and the other forty, and both had children. Also, both were divorced. They had moved to Los Angeles a year apart in the early 1910s. Although they had both migrated from Italy, one had originally moved to New York in the early 1900s while the other had moved directly to Los Angeles. Both of these women recorded attending over twenty births in 1917. Their affidavits suggest that they worked together to cover community needs. In April and September, in particular, the two midwives frequently worked on alternate days.

Three Japanese midwives submitted information for 1917. Two of these worked in the city while one worked exclusively in the county. The two that attended cases in the city were of similar ages, late to mid-thirties, but the woman who worked for the county was older, almost fifty. All were married but, unlike the Italian and French midwives, none of these women had children. Of the two women working in the city, one could speak and read English, the other could do so only a little, while the woman in the county did not speak or read any English. The latter had moved to Los Angeles in the late 1900s, while the two working in the city had moved to Los Angeles in the early 1910s. All three moved directly from Japan to Los Angeles. The two women in the city lived quite close to each other, and the evidence suggests that these women also worked as colleagues. Similar to the Italian midwives, these two attended to cases on alternate days.

The stories of these women testify to the strength of midwifery despite the longtime efforts by physicians and nurses in the city to replace or remove it from the medical landscape. Unlike their former counterparts, however, the majority of these women possessed diplomas. The state's attempts at regulation had created a space within which women could continue the practice of midwifery in the city. Yet their ethnicity, particularly in the case of the Japanese, also continued to raise questions about their assimilability.

Under financial pressure during the Great Depression, the city slated the termination of the obstetrics division for June 1, 1933. They took this action despite the evident need for the program. The number of women attended to by the division slowly increased in the 1910s from 263 in 1915 to 495 in 1919 and then rose dramatically in the 1920s to approximately 1,300 annually. In its last year within the health department (1933), the division delivered 1,687 babies, which constituted 10 percent of all births in the city.[86] Feeling increasingly intense pressure from female reformers, religious organizations, and concerned citizens, the city government devised monthly fixes to the financial problem while seeking a long-term solution.[87]

Community members voiced strong opposition to the elimination of the program. Approximately one hundred members of the Plymouth Congregational Church suggested transferring the service to the county welfare department to secure the necessary funds.[88] The Los Angeles Forum argued to cut other departments' budgets so that the service could continue unaltered.[89] The board of health commissioners pleaded with the city council, emphasizing the diversity of groups who had expressed their support for the program: "Gentlemen of the Council, you have heard the voice of the community from every women's group, including Jewish welfare, Catholic welfare, and Protestant welfare. . . . In the name of God and for humanity, we call upon you to provide."[90] Over five hundred female members of the various metropolitan Methodist Episcopal churches signed a petition declaring that "abandonment of such service rendered our underprivileged motherhood and future childhood would be an appalling tragedy to very many destitute women. Its continuation is not merely opportune. It is imperative."[91] Finally, the Friday Morning Club, the Los Angeles District Parent-Teachers Association, the Ebell Club, Children's Hospital Society, Los Angeles League of Women Voters, Council of Catholic Women, Council of Jewish Women, United Church Women of Los Angeles, Association of Volunteers in Social Service, Catholic Woman's Club, and the Catholic Big Sisters signed a joint petition. In addition to financial, practical, and moral arguments, these women's organizations articulated a concern directly related to the Great Depression: "We can not neglect the mothers in the families of the unemployed, nor can we afford to jeopardize the health of our future citizens."[92]

These petitions played no small part in eventually convincing the Los Angeles County Charities Department to take over the service at the end of the year.[93] Facing scarce city revenues and this vocal citizenry, the city looked to state law. Officials interpreted state law in such a way as to argue that the county should pay for the service. They believed that "state law clearly places the burden upon the counties." The county initially responded, however, that it did not have the money. Moreover, it argued that "the city having conducted these services over a long period of years, had a moral if not legal obligation to continue to do so."[94] Still, on December 20, 1933, the county formally took over the program.

While limited in service, the city health department's division of obstetrics provided a unique solution to a public health question. Whether or not Los Angeles had a high infant-mortality rate in comparison to other cities did not lessen public health providers' interest in lowering those figures. The "midwife" problem was a metaphor as well as a response to the growing number of immigrants at the turn of the century whose ethnicity and race differed greatly from their predecessors. Maude Foster Weston first addressed the issue by creating a specialized public health nursing position: the maternity nurse. She also aided the city in attempting to regulate midwifery by instructing public health nurses to ferret out offenders, a role they continued to play once the city absorbed the program into the health department. The city built on Weston's tactics of replacement and regulation by creating stricter laws and providing prenatal as well as postnatal health care. Moreover, by literally delivering the city's children, the city augmented the breadth of Weston's already broad vision of public health. By extending its reach into private homes to perform one of the most intimate of matters, the city expanded the scope of its public health services. Still, these services were taken in part from the very women the city was trying to supplant: midwives. In this way the city and Weston responded to the expectations of the women to whom they were trying to render health services.

Chapter 5

The Challenge of Constructing Venereal Disease Programs

Physician Etta C. Jeancon worked for the Los Angeles city health department's venereal disease division during World War I. In her annual report of activities in June 1919, Jeancon recounted various attempts by female prisoners to use the courts to "test ... the scope" of the city's public health powers to arrest the spread of syphilis and gonorrhea.[1] In particular, women contested the city's physical exam, quarantine, and treatment of their bodies in the name of patriotism. Jeancon told stories of women presenting scientific evidence of their purity, of claiming mistaken identity, and of outright refusal to allow their bodies to be examined.

Citing an instance that took place approximately one year after the United States declared war on Germany, Jeancon described in detail one woman's refusal to submit to a physical. Arrested for vagrancy and lewdness, the woman justified her position based on the fact that "aside from imbibing a bit she was a respectable woman." In the eyes of the police, health officials, and female reformers, however, alcoholism and prostitution were mutually dependent activities. Although Jeancon did not immediately press the issue, she also did not consent to the woman's release. In response, the woman's lawyer requested a writ of habeas corpus. In the ensuing proceedings, the court denied the accused's appeal for liberation. Instead it ruled that "the testimony showed that the woman was guilty of lewd conduct, that [the health department was] justified in having reason to believe that she was infected, that the public must be protected from the spread of venereal disease, and that the spirit of the law rather than the letter should be interpreted here." Although Jeancon had not yet attempted to force the woman to yield her body to an exam, the court found that the physician was "justified in pursuing such a course."

The court sent the woman back to jail, and it must have seemed to health department officials that questions about their power over this woman's body were settled. Yet this woman persisted in refusing to allow health officials to examine her for another six months. Jeancon left the reason for the woman's change in stance unrecorded, stating only that she "gave her consent, was examined, found positive for gonorrhea, and sent to the Los Feliz Hospital." At Los Feliz—the city's detention/treatment center for women diagnosed with syphilis and/or gonorrhea—this woman spent approximately five weeks receiving daily douches and topical medication to eliminate her infection. She was finally released after completing this treatment. Yet she did not enjoy her freedom for long. Jeancon's final statement about this case was the following: "It is interesting to note that this woman has since been arrested again and is again at the Los Feliz Hospital for similar infection."

Jeancon's anecdote became part of the public record. She offered this story as proof of the struggles endured by the health department in carrying out its venereal disease programs. Because of the nature of syphilis and gonorrhea's transmission, policies toward curbing these ailments turned private bedrooms into places subject to public oversight. Health officials justified their actions because they believed that preventing the spread of venereal disease through whatever means they deemed necessary was more important than the rights of any single individual. They were not alone in this belief, nor was the curtailment of civil liberties in this historical period isolated to issues of health.[2] At the same time, Jeancon's report is illuminating in other ways that perhaps the health department did not intend. Although Jeancon's preservation of the woman's anonymity obscures what we know about her, Jeancon's paraphrasing of her defense provides evidence of dissent and negotiation. While the health department had the power to force an exam, they paused in exercising this authority. Thus, as other scholars have shown, even within the criminal justice system, inmates found ways to exert some control over their situation.[3]

California led the nation in changing public health policies toward venereal disease.[4] In 1911, state officials made syphilis and gonorrhea reportable diseases. In 1914, Los Angeles city officials passed an ordinance empowering the health department to quarantine individuals with syphilis and gonorrhea. This local law, however, only applied to women who had been convicted of crimes of prostitution and vagrancy. In 1917, as part of World War I mobilization efforts, the California legislature authorized city health officials throughout the state to isolate anyone—men and women—whom they suspected of being infectious. This modification allowed the health department to examine all persons upon their arrest rather than waiting for a conviction. While the law was neutral as to sex, in Los Angeles the law's execution disproportionately affected women. In 1919, officials quarantined 96.5 percent of the women they found infected with venereal disease but only 49 percent of the men they found infected.[5]

Differential public health policy accounted for part of the discrepancy. In his annual report for 1919, Arthur Rogers, director of the city's venereal disease division, explained this difference by saying "that it [was] possible that the examiner for women was more persistent in her efforts to secure a positive finding before reporting her case as negative."[6] He also suggested that "it must be apparent to anyone who gives attention to these things that a larger proportion of [Jeancon's] examinations were of individuals who make a business of prostitution, than was true among men." In addition, health officials consistently released "noninfectious" gonorrheal men if they promised to seek treatment at the city's voluntary clinic. Although the city sponsored a similar clinic for women, it did not afford them the same option until 1922. Despite the disproportion, Rogers insisted that the "strictness" within which treatment was carried out within the quarantined areas was equal.

War, prostitution, and venereal disease are three subjects often studied in conjunction with one another. Historians argue that World War I transformed public health campaigns against venereal disease.[7] Certainly city health officials in Los Angeles were emboldened by the increased financial support from the state of California and by public concern over the high rates of venereal disease among the army's new inductees. The war allowed the city to purchase the necessary equipment for the Wasserman test, to expand its genito-urinary clinic for men, open a women's voluntary clinic, and to create an involuntary treatment center (Los Feliz Hospital) for women accused of prostitution and vagrancy. But rather than causing fundamental changes in the way that local public health campaigns against venereal disease were carried out, these changes were more a matter of scale than scope.

Female reformers laid out an agenda for the eradication of venereal disease when they attempted to eliminate vice from the city at the turn of the twentieth century. Unlike their experience with milk, where they struggled to advance their authority through science, or nursing, where their use of maternalism went largely unchallenged, venereal disease programs allowed female reformers to synergize strategies of science and sympathy. The creation of Los Feliz Hospital fulfilled a long-standing goal of the social hygiene movement: the creation of a separate institution to treat women's physical ailments and provide moral guidance. It was an action that should be seen as an extension of turn-of-the-century movements throughout the nation to create feminist structures within which to monitor young women's sexuality.[8] At the same time, the records documenting reformers' work provide evidence of the responses of red-light district sex workers to their changing relationship with the local state.[9] In the end, everyday negotiations between prostitutes, women accused of prostitution, reformers, and city officials shaped public health policy.

Throughout the late nineteenth and early twentieth centuries, physicians in Los Angeles repeatedly complained about the persistence of gonorrhea and syphilis among the city's population. One physician went so far as to claim that gonorrhea "often furnishe[d] the young doctor his first case and the old physician his last patient."[10] European scientists identified the microbes that caused gonorrhea in 1885 and syphilis in 1905. Building on these discoveries, Augustus Paul von Wasserman developed a diagnostic blood test for syphilis in 1906, and four years later, in 1910, Paul Ehrlich discovered the "magic bullet" to cure syphilis, an arsenic compound he patented under the name Salvarsan. In Los Angeles, these changes in medical knowledge and diagnostics did not go unnoticed by health officials and the local medical community, but they did not automatically change their medical practices. For instance, health officials shied away from Salvarsan because its application was long, expensive, and proved deadly if not administered by a very experienced hand. And, they did not immediately purchase the equipment necessary for conducting Wasserman tests because it was expensive. In addition, no specific cure existed for treating gonorrhea until the 1930s.

Until 1911, California did not require private physicians or health officials to report cases of venereal disease. In that year, state senator James B. Holohan sponsored a bill that added venereal diseases to a list of contagious diseases that all coroners, health officials, and private physicians were required to file a written report with the state board of health for each case they encountered.[11] Presumably because of the sordid connotations associated with venereal disease, the code specified that in these specific cases the patient's name should be omitted from the record and replaced with a number. Despite this precaution to preserve patient privacy, neither private physicians nor health officials were eager to comply with the law. In fact, seven years later the California State Board of Health admitted that they rarely enforced compulsory reporting.[12]

Despite the reticence of officials to take more aggressive action, other groups were ready to proceed. Social hygiene was a national movement that emerged from semiorganized disparate local actions against vice in the late nineteenth century. It emphasized that prostitution degraded the family. Social hygienists viewed venereal disease as a symptom, not the cause of this social contagion. The eradication of prostitution, the suppression of urban vice, and the promotion of male self-restraint became the aims of this new movement, while the arrest of venereal disease became one of its effects. Clubwomen and members of the social hygiene movement worked together to attack vice in California in ways that impacted municipal control over venereal disease. Social hygienists made use of medical knowledge by repeatedly citing the impact on women's health as a primary reason to curb vice. Left untreated, syphilis and gonorrhea could cause sterility, threaten the health of fetuses both in vitro and during birth, produce internal damage to vascular and nervous systems, and in some cases result in death. In 1919, the health commissioner of Los Angeles, L. M. Powers, "estimated that not less than 70% of the operations performed on women [were] caused by" complications of gonorrhea.[13]

The social hygiene movement enjoyed particular legislative success (legislative success as distinct from actually creating a vice-free society) in Los Angeles, in particular, and California, in general. In Los Angeles, the social hygiene movement drew its support from a strong women's rights movement and there was overlap between participants. In 1902, citizens of Los Angeles attempted to transform the city's social environment by prohibiting gambling and prostitution.[14] Bolstered by the federal government's passage of the Mann Act in 1910 and the passage of women's suffrage in California in 1911, Los Angeles adopted "The Rooming-House Ordinance" on May 13, 1912, declaring it illegal for any person to use a rooming house, lodging house, or hotel within the city for the purpose of having sexual intercourse with a person to whom he or she was not married.[15] Armed with suffrage, the following year Los Angelenas took their anti-vice agenda to the state legislature and helped secure the passage of the Red-Light Abatement Act of 1913.[16]

The Red-Light Abatement Act deemed houses of prostitution to be "nuisances" and granted "any citizen, whether personally damaged or not, to bring action." If the court found the residence in violation of the law, it issued a fine against the property and prohibited the estate from being used as a bawdy house in the future. While the act did not directly mention venereal disease, it attacked what these reformers perceived as its source: brothels. As Rose Bullard said, speaking before the female members of the Friday Morning Club in April 1910 in a talk entitled "The Social Evil: Its Menace to the Home," "The prophylaxis of venereal disease and the prevention of prostitution are indissolubly linked. We cannot dissociate the effect from the cause."[17] In Los Angeles, a newly formed Morals Efficiency Association quickly took action and facilitated a shutdown of the vice district. Prostitution, according to a contemporary, was not entirely eliminated, however. Instead, it was only reduced to a minimum. Not all women's groups agreed with the Moral Efficiency Association's tactics. In 1917, the association embarked on a fund-raising campaign and in their circular asked people "to report to the association any violation of the Law governing morals ... confidential complaints received." According to the *Los Angeles Times*, some women's groups objected because they wanted reformers to focus on education and rehabilitation efforts instead of "snooping."[18]

The Red-Light Abatement Act strengthened the resolve of public health officials in Los Angeles to take a more public stance to abate the spread of venereal disease in the city. Although the state law required physicians to report cases, it did not obligate cities to publish those statistics. Los Angeles began publicizing the prevalence of venereal disease in 1914, the year after the passage of the Red-Light Abatement Act. In this first year, however, the city reported a mere 364 cases of venereal disease. In response to those numbers, chief health commissioner Luther M. Powers wrote, "obviously a very small percentage of existing cases are reported."[19] Turn-of-the-century epidemiologists estimated that infection rates for syphilis among the public ranged from 10 to 25 percent and they put gonorrhea rates even higher.[20] Because the population in Los Angeles exceeded 300,000, Powers assumed that the city's statistics presented an inaccurate picture of venereal disease in the city. While Powers believed that physicians were not complying with the law, he found it difficult to prove. Furthermore, the state code did not provide for punitive measures and thereby limited his ability to enforce the statute.

Perhaps out of frustration, or perhaps out of practicality, or perhaps both, the city health department turned its attention to the one group it believed it could control: prostitutes. In 1914, Los Angeles passed an ordinance obligating the health department to examine all women for venereal disease who were convicted of "the offense of vagrancy," or for being "a lewd or dissolute person," or for "living in or about a house of ill-fame, or of keeping or residing in a house of ill-fame, or of soliciting or offering her body for the purpose of prostitution, or the violation of any other law ordinance of which the evidence shows the defendant is guilty of an act or acts of prostitution."[21] If the exam yielded positive results, the health commissioner was empowered to "immediately remove such person so affected to some hospital or place designated by the City Council of the City, that such person shall be there held and be given treatment for such disease until the said person has fully recovered, or until such disease has reached a non-communicable stage." Members of the local medical community supported this action, calling it an "excellent" means to "lessen the venereal infections" in the city. They also viewed this as a means to provide "a most unfortunate class of women" with access to treatment.

The year 1914 was not the first time that the city exercised medical power over incarcerated bodies. Since 1903, the city regularly inspected the bodies of juveniles for venereal disease. In that year, the city set up a juvenile court and soon after its creation appointed a physician to conduct a physical exam of all male youth upon their remand. Depending on the determination of physician J. A. Colliver, the boys were treated for conditions that he deemed a source for their "incorrigible" behavior. This included "the removal of tonsils and adenoids, relief of a physmosis by circumcision or retraction, [and] relief of abnormal conditions of the teeth." At first the city did not subject every girl to a similar exam. This policy changed in July 1912, when the Juvenile Court ruled that "every girl brought to the court must be completely examined, and a medical report of each case be given to Judge Curtis D. Wilbur before the case was tried."[22] As a consequence of this ruling, girls were subjected to a test even before the judge had determined the disposition of the case. In examining the bodies of juveniles, the physicians in charge more often found girls rather than boys to be infected. Olga McNeile, the Medical Probation Officer of the Los Angeles Juvenile Court, attributed the difference in rates to the fact that "the majority of the girls who come under the jurisdiction of the Juvenile Court are arrested for sexual crimes. This element does not enter so strongly into the boys who come under the Court."[23] McNeile's comment is important for understanding the extent to which the city's focus during World War I on women to arrest the spread of venereal disease was in many ways unexceptional given its previous policies that were based on a gendered view of whom to arrest for what type of crime.

Although the city health department appeared resolved to take action, its attempt to run a campaign against venereal disease prior to the war was limited. In particular, although the city had the power to examine, detain, and treat women for venereal disease who were held in its city's jails, there is no evidence that it actually used this power.[24] In retrospect, the main constraint appears to have been financial.[25] The city's stance began to change in 1917. In that year, the Los Angeles Society of Social Hygiene and the Los Angeles Health Department held a series of conferences to discuss the nature of venereal disease. They pressed the city council to fund a municipal clinic as a response to the number of syphilitic men who dominated the city's statistics. In the first year in which the city publicized its records, men constituted 76 percent of all syphilitic cases reported and 64 percent of all venereal disease cases reported.[26] Establishing a men's voluntary clinic reflected the sentiment that men, as husbands and fathers, owed a responsibility to their families to seek treatment if they could not curb their impulses. The lobby succeeded and the Genito-Urinary Clinic opened its doors on February 23, 1917, and, suiting the needs of its working-class clientele, maintained hours every Tuesday and Friday from

7 P.M. to 8 P.M. Ironically, for a program responding to vice, the only space they could acquire was four small rooms located above a popular pool hall.[27]

According to Alfred R. Rogers, the clinic's original supervisor, curing those patients who walked through its door was his first goal. Using education to prevent the spread of venereal disease was his second. He believed that the poor, whom he considered the "worst disseminators" of venereal disease, were "not so vicious as they are ignorant."[28] Rogers stressed the importance of verbal instructions as well as the necessity for "terse, easily understood literature" that detailed the seriousness of the disease, its contagious nature, and the "fallacy of self-treatment and of treatment by quacks and charlatans."[29] He also established a "bulletin board" in the clinic waiting rooms to educate in a nonobtrusive manner.

At the clinic, patients received a physical exam. If Rogers suspected a case of syphilis, he instructed the patient to report to the city laboratory to have his or her blood drawn. While the city bacteriologist, Placida Gardner, limited these visits to Wednesdays and less than a dozen cases were sent in the clinic's initial four months, she complained that "a large amount of time [was] used up in doing" the test. Gardner found that these time restraints "compelled" the laboratory "to limit the work to those patients who [were] sent from the clinics officially connected with the health department" instead of making their diagnostic capabilities available to "all patients not able to pay for the test elsewhere."[30]

Rogers's concern with quackery suggests the popularity of alternative medical treatment for venereal disease. Patients might have been reticent to attend the clinic for a number of reasons, including the therapies involved. Salvarsan, an arsenic-based compound, had become the standard treatment for syphilis since Paul Ehrlich publicized his discovery of it in 1910.[31] Physicians who subscribed to the local medical journal, the *Southern California Practitioner*, would have been aware of the debates over the benefits and risks of using Salvarsan. The journal reprinted information from *Pediatrics*, the *Journal of the American Medical Association* (*JAMA*), and included reprints that appeared in *JAMA* from Spanish, German, and British medical journals. All of the excerpts indicated enthusiasm for the new cure, especially given the alternative of mercury. According to *JAMA*, "There [was] scarcely a patient who does not become depressed, anemic, and lose weight under mercurial treatment."[32] Still, the writers of these early reports reserved the right to pass final judgment once the drug was marketed. In particular, *JAMA*'s editors warned that other arsenic-based drugs had proven to be of mixed benefit due to the "toxic effects of arsenic."[33] Two years later, as reports of fatalities appeared in the press, the

Southern California Practitioner printed articles that attempted to assure local physicians of Salvarsan's safety. Printing editorials from *JAMA*, local physicians were told that fatalities were due either to negligent patients, physicians, or in the case of one woman, of complications due to a combination of an advanced stage of syphilis and pregnancy.[34] Given the fatalities and the technical nature of administering Salvarsan, it is not surprising that there was some hesitance to its use. Consequently, taking mercury either orally, in salves, or in vapors continued to play a key role in treatment. Admittedly, this was not without some danger. Yet, many physicians found it to be worth the risk. In 1912, two years after the advent of Salvarsan, the editors of the *Southern California Practitioner* cautioned its readers not to abandon mercury:

> While the use of Salvarsan often produces favorable results where mercury has failed, yet it is quite definitely shaping itself into the fact that instead of supplanting mercury and iodine, Salvarsan is invaluably supplementing them in certain manifestations of the disease, and that when properly used in combination with the older treatment, it offers the most adequate means of treating syphilis.[35]

Patients who submitted to these remedies did find relief and, consequently, many stopped attending the clinics long before physicians considered them cured. Mona Bettin, who worked in the women's division, said "many of the patients promptly leave town after being released from [Los Feliz Hospital] and since they are in better health than they have been for some time, they keep putting off the continuation of their treatment until the far distant future."[36] According to Alfred R. Rogers, "few of [the male ex-cons] ever find their way to the clinic, though all promise to come" and instead "a majority of these men leave the city shortly after their release."[37] Jeancon's account of her experience at the city's voluntary clinic concurred with that of her colleagues: "Our records show that 111 cases [out of 178] failed to return. Some were turned over to other physicians for treatment; some were lost sight of completely. A great many of the latter are old syphilitics who imagine they are well because they have no active manifestations."[38] All of Rogers's, Bettin's, and Jeancon's accounts express exasperation. Their responses, however, differed based upon their genders. Whereas Arthur Rogers described attempts to conduct follow-ups as "more or less futile," Etta Jeancon found "the social worker has been a great aid in bringing in delinquent patients."[39] Their expectations about the role of the state in fostering everyday medical relations helped elicit different responses; female reformers in Los Angeles had long used the state to enter homes in order to sway women into using the city's health care services.

The issue of continued treatment posed a major problem for health officials. Officials focused on treating symptoms rather than the root of the disease because curing syphilis was complicated and no "magic bullet" existed for gonorrhea. Health officials forced patients to undergo treatment only until they considered them noninfectious rather than cured. This helps to explain why the woman in the opening vignette found herself back so quickly at Los Feliz Hospital. Gonorrheal patients needed to produce two smears within forty-eight hours that did not have bacteria present. Officials judged syphilis patients as noninfectious when all of their lesions of the skin or mucous membranes healed. Despite knowing that allopathic medical treatments were arduous, Rogers steadfastly continued to blame alternative medicine for patients' reticence. He believed that patients' unorthodox experiences made them reluctant to attend the clinics. He contended that "many have been bled by unscrupulous charlatans, masquerading under the names of physician, until they have lost all confidence in the ability and honesty of the medical profession and have become convinced that their disease is incurable."[40] This threat to official programs and powers incited the health department to continue its attempts to rid the city of alternative care.

Although the clinic opened a month before the United States officially entered World War I, it would owe much of its success to this conflict. The voluntary clinic remained an essential part of the city's venereal-disease program for the next decade. Rogers saw the clinic as a means to promote the city's public health reputation as both an innovator and as a model of success. He proudly noted, in 1917, that the Los Angeles clinic was only one of six operating nationwide and he believed that it could "be made one of the largest and most beneficial institutions in the West."[41] Yet, while the numbers attending the clinic grew and its hours increased, much to Rogers's chagrin, the small number of staff members remained constant. The city employed one full-time and one part-time physician, a clerk, and a steward to work in the men's clinics. While finances affected staffing, Rogers's adherence to Victorian ethics also limited the city's venereal disease programs. Rogers believed in only hiring "medical men" to assist him in the clinic. Unfortunately for him, male medical students had little interest in this field. According to Rogers, the college clinics presented the students with "interesting" and "instructive" cases while, in comparison, the work at the venereal disease clinic seemed mundane.[42] While costlier, Rogers eventually hired an assistant rather than rely on temporary student volunteers.[43]

World War I transformed public health campaigns against venereal disease. City health officials in Los Angeles were emboldened by the increased financial support from the state of California and by the high rates of venereal disease among new inductees.⁴⁴ The draft revealed without a doubt the prevalence of syphilis and gonorrhea in the United States. After tallying the numbers, the military found that infection rates ranged from 13 to 25 percent and that over 80 percent of new troops had contracted venereal disease before arriving for duty.⁴⁵ This finding surprised the public, who still tacitly believed that venereal disease could only spread among the "immoral." Exposing the endemic and indiscriminate nature of venereal disease generated support for public health programs for suppression and prevention.

At the state and municipal levels, Californians designed a specific apparatus to respond to this public health crisis before the federal government did. The state established a Bureau of Social Hygiene on August 13, 1917, and the governor appropriated $30,000 for two years. According to the secretary of the State Board of Health, Los Angeles led the state in its local efforts. Within months, the city approved a plan to spend $25,000 on controlling the spread of venereal disease.⁴⁶ Both of these actions were taken prior to the federal government's passage of the Chamberlain-Kahn Act in July 1918. California, Oregon, and Washington had a significant impact on this legislation, since many of those involved with successful local programs in these western states were directly concerned with its passage.⁴⁷ The federal government intended to assist, not to supplant, efforts already underway throughout the United States. The Chamberlain-Kahn Act established an Interdepartmental Social Hygiene Board and a special venereal disease division within the United States Public Health Service (USPHS). The board was given funds to allocate to states for detention centers; however, the application of these funds was extremely limited. The USPHS funneled federal funds throughout the country but their administration remained in the hands of local officials.

In sum, the war provided Los Angeles with the resources it needed to develop a comprehensive municipal venereal disease program. On top of funding, the California Military Welfare Commission helped the city undertake a publicity campaign. Judging by the major jump in number of cases reported by private physicians, from 471 in 1917 to 1,867 in 1919, these efforts seemed effective. Additionally, state officials amended the state code to expand local officials' power for the purpose of suppressing venereal disease. In 1917, the state gave local officials "full powers of inspection, examination, isolation, and disinfection of all persons, places, and things." This power extended to any person that the health department could "reasonably" suspect as being infectious. The state enabled local authorities to establish isolation centers, and to hold persons until officials no longer considered them "a menace to the health of the city."⁴⁸

The war also had an impact on treatment. Besides the possible complications of using Salvarsan, it was also expensive. Prior to the war the drug was patented and produced by a German firm. The onset of war in Europe disrupted distribution to American markets, contributing to Salvarsan's scarcity and expense. With the official entrance of the United States into the war, the Federal Trade Commission decided that it would not be a violation of international trade to allow three American pharmaceutical companies to produce what had been patented as "Salvarsan" as "Arsphenamine." What cost $4 per dose before the war, and which had risen to $35 in some places, was reduced to no more than $1.50 per dose.[49] Increased access and the drop in price allowed the city health department to increase its use of this drug. In 1918, the city administered 17 treatments of Salvarsan to 7 men and 270 treatments to 140 women. The following year the city administered 94 treatments of Arsphenamine to 35 men and 642 treatments of Arsphenamine to 200 women.[50]

The war, however, did not seem to change the public health strategies for treating gonorrhea. The mainstay of the health department's treatment for women was to prescribe a douche. In Los Feliz's first year, the city administered over 10,000 douches to the two hundred women who entered this institution. The volume of these treatments led to interesting consequences. In 1918, the city engineer was brought in to study "the discharge of sewage into cesspools which [were] located in the property across from the road from said hospital."[51] He determined that "due to the large amount of water discharged from said hospital, and to the nature of the soil," the city needed to build a sewer.

In discussing attempts at treating and curtailing venereal disease among women, the city's conversations between 1918 and 1920 focused on gonorrheal patients. As Mona Bettin, the supervisor of Los Feliz Hospital, remarked, "The greater number of these women had gonorrheal infection—that disease which is so difficult to eradicate and which taxes our patience to the utmost."[52] Without a cure, gonorrheal symptoms returned and women ended up being rearrested, reincarcerated, and retreated for venereal disease. The health department only discussed this seemingly never-ending cycle in relation to women.

The focus on protecting or redeeming women's sexuality was part of the longer history of reforms regarding white slavery, age of consent laws, and blood tests for marriage, which were all part of a larger movement for women's rights in the late nineteenth and early twentieth centuries. What had become different was the potential scale of the problem of policing sexuality in a time of war. According to law enforcement records, the army and navy stationed approximately five thousand soldiers and sailors within Los Angeles and thousands more in nearby camps. "Following them," the police contended, "came those who lure toward vice."[53] Although the city had theoretically limited the numbers of opportunities for vice, just across city limits the county's incorporated towns seemed to be taking advantage of their independence by allowing dance halls, gambling, and other industries of vice to flourish. Social reformers theorized that this situation led to the spread of venereal disease as these businesses "attracted thousands of pleasure-loving and often irresponsible transients who spend their money and drive away."[54] Moreover, the California State Board of Health claimed that "at least a third of all women who [gave] their bodies for immoral purposes [were] suffering from some form of venereal disease." Their study included "not merely professional prostitutes, but other girls and young women who, to satisfy their love of finery, to eke out a scanty income or for other reasons, occasionally lapse from virtue."[55] Women across the nation became the focus of venereal suppression efforts. In Los Angeles, these women found themselves incarcerated at the Los Feliz Hospital.

During World War I, the city developed different types of facilities for men and women. The city made space within its East Side jail for treating men but procured a separate and specialized space—a place it named Los Feliz Hospital—to detain and treat women.[56] The formation of government sponsored

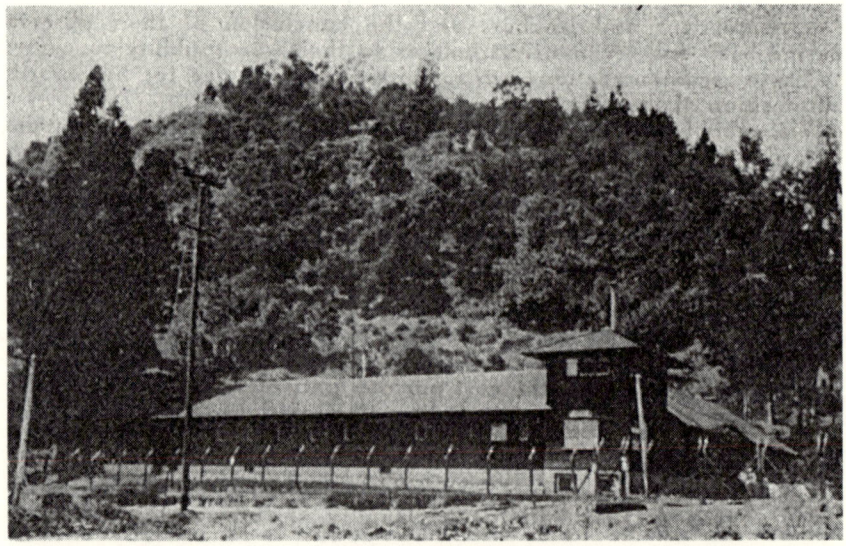

Figure 6 Los Feliz Hospital, "Nestled on the Northern Slopes of Elysian Park."
(Source: *Public Health: A Monthly Bulletin of the Los Angeles City Health Department* 5, no 7 [1918], 7. History and Special Collections Division, Louise M. Darling, Biomedical Library, UCLA)

detention centers for women was central to federal mobilization efforts.[57] Like San Diego, San Francisco, Portland, and Seattle, Los Angeles designed a specific apparatus to respond to this public health crisis before the federal government did. The city approved a plan to spend $25,000 on controlling the spread of venereal disease, which included establishing Los Feliz Hospital.[58]

Opened on January 28, 1918, Los Feliz Hospital was located at 1450 Los Feliz Road, a remote area that bordered Elysian Park northeast of downtown Los Angeles.[59] Its isolated nature was accentuated by the fact that the nearest streetcar line was a mile away. The building accommodated fifty to sixty female inmates. The city enclosed the facility with a wire fence that was connected to an electric alarm system. The staff consisted of a nonresident woman physician, a live-in female supervisor, a vocational teacher appointed by the Board of Education, three nurses, a cook, and three guards.[60] In addition to this staff, the city appointed a six-woman advisory Board of Social Workers to watch over Los Feliz's rehabilitation programs. These women were not licensed social workers but, instead, well-known clubwomen who were married to civic leaders. Rose Baruch, the head of the advisory board, was also the vice president of the Los Angeles Social Hygiene Association.[61] These women wanted to ensure that Los Feliz would not just accomplish health officials' goals of suppression but realize their own ideas about prevention. As members of the social hygiene movement, they believed that a double standard of criminal justice existed that resulted in the victimization of women—both wives and red-light-district sex workers—and that providing money for treatment and vocational training would correct this imbalance.

The average age of women incarcerated at Los Feliz was twenty-six. The city classified these women as prostitutes, drunks, and drug addicts and provided very little information that would make their individual identities discernable. Baruch remarked in a report to the health department that "in this shifting population, every race, creed, color, and condition have been represented, white, yellow, black, and even the red people, having been a part of the motley assemblage."[62] Her comment correlates with the police records from the mid-1920s, which suggest that the city arrested approximately 60 to 70 percent white women, 15 to 25 percent African American women, and 10 to 15 percent Mexican women for this type of offense.[63] Health officials, thus, did not associate venereal disease with any particular ethnicity or race. They did, however, correlate it with a particular social group: single working-class women. Baruch believed that most of these women were "old offenders before the law." Yet she also determined that a number were new "delinquents produced by the war exigencies."[64] Health officials originally believed that many of these cases would be "feeble-minded" women, but their experience did not confirm that preconception. Mona Bettin, the female physician in charge of treatment at Los Feliz, argued that the majority of women could not be considered medically unsound, just "weak-minded and lack[ing] in will power."[65] Bettin believed that these women would be best served by an industrial home where she thought they could reorganize their lives instead of continuing to go "around in a circle . . . yield[ing] to temptation, get[ting] into trouble and out again."

A woman's journey to Los Feliz began at the city's central jail, where a female physician representing the city health department administered a blood test and conducted a visual exam. If the accused tested positive or exhibited physical symptoms, officials brought the woman to Los Feliz in a police car and, immediately upon arrival, subjected her to a bath and hair treatment for eliminating and protecting against lice. The department then issued her institutional clothing and took her personal belongings away to be fumigated. This process implied that public health reformers viewed venereal disease as an all-encompassing contagion. Speaking to the Friday Morning Club in 1910, physician Rose Bullard had contended that venereal diseases could be contracted through kissing, shaking hands, sharing utensils, linen, and drinking cups.[66] These actions perhaps also reflected their knowledge of the jails. The city completed the experience by severely limiting visitors whom health officials feared would bring "opiates" and tobacco.[67]

The advisory board's beliefs about labor guided the rehabilitative process at Los Feliz. Health officials theorized that prisoners should not be allowed to idle, arguing that if patients' "hands were busy their minds would be less full of gossip and mischief."[68] By mischief, health officials were perhaps referring to the number of schemes for escaping the premises that patients managed successfully to concoct and deploy. In the first four months, eighteen women (22 percent) navigated around the nurses, guards, and electric-alarmed wire fence to gain their freedom. Clippings from the *Los Angeles Times* provide a better sense of how women accomplished this feat.[69] In 1919, May Jonson, Anna Nelson, Helen Mason, May Goins, and Irene Garner used "a pair of shears and butcher knife" to cut a hole in the fence while everyone else was otherwise engaged in dinner. In 1921, Georgia Stanley's exit "baffled county authorities." According to the *Los Angeles Times* three men pulled up in a car, walked through the gate, picked up the "handsome blonde," put her in the car and drove away. Although the guard "gave chase," he was "soon outdistanced." The paper asked, "Was she kidnapped [or] rescued?" In 1927, Grace Kenney, whom the police arrested "for masquerading in male attire," managed to hoist herself over the eight-foot-high fence. Patients' desire to leave did not completely puzzle Los Feliz's managers. They immediately responded by decreasing the average treatment from ten to five weeks. In comparison to Adam Hodges's findings about Portland's detention center or Nancy Bristow's descriptions of the centers sponsored by the Commission on Training Camp Activities, this action made women's imprisonment at Los Feliz markedly brief.[70] In spite of these changes, women still fled. Altogether, 12 percent broke out of quarantine the first year, and "escaped" remained a statistical category throughout Los Feliz's history.

In response to officials' desires for ways to maintain order and their own beliefs about rehabilitation, the advisory board convinced the Board of Education to appoint two teachers to instruct the inmates in "elementary school work, gardening, sewing, and other occupational activities."[71] During the war, Bettin also included "patriotic talks" and learning the Pledge of Allegiance as part of this training. In addition, an Episcopal diocese held a weekly service. Comparable tasks at San Francisco's Arequipa Sanatorium for working-class women suffering from tuberculosis bore little resemblance to the actual types of jobs these women might have searched for upon release.[72] A similar point might be made about the activities at Los Feliz. The average length of incarceration—five to six weeks—did not allow for any in-depth job training that might have yielded greater occupational mobility. Furthermore, in at least one aspect the activities were outright exploitative. By furnishing the hospital with workers to mend and sew the garments worn by the inmates, the sheets they slept on, and the curtains on the windows, this "vocational training" helped mitigate the costs of running the institution. Still, the advisory board truly believed that these activities served as gateways to domestic labor and garment factory positions.

Toward that end, in 1919 one member of the advisory board asked the city to permit her to provide the patients with the opportunity to earn some money by making clothes during their stay at Los Feliz. The request bounced back and forth between the health commissioner, the city council's health and sanitation committee, the city attorney, and the city council for a month and a half. The city attorney quickly determined that no legal barrier prevented women from working for private parties and receiving compensation. A delay arose, however, when the city council raised a concern that venereal disease could be transmitted via the handling of clothing. Once the health commissioner, L. M. Powers, assured the city council that there was no threat, the city approved the plan.[73] These women were allowed to work but it did not serve as a way out of quarantine. Instead, the health department's beliefs about these women's susceptibility to vice and the emphasis on stemming venereal disease during World War I prompted them to keep these women in isolation until it no longer considered them a menace to the public's health.

Outside of work and a decreased average time of treatment, how could the female managers of Los Feliz persuade its residents to comply? The city health department turned to the courts. On March 27, 1918, police arrested a woman, described by Jeancon as a "white prostitute and morphine fiend," for vagrancy and sent her to Los Feliz after she tested positive for gonorrhea.[74] The woman escaped the next day. On April 30, police arrested her again, but she used a different name. The judge sentenced her to thirty days. She again tested positive for gonorrhea but, because Los Feliz could not accommodate all of the women who were found positive, she received her treatment in the Central Jail. Health officials learned her identity during these thirty days but waited until the end of her sentence to serve her with a warrant for breaking her previous quarantine. In court, she argued that she was not the same offender, but the health department contended that they "easily established" her identity. The department persuaded the judge to sentence her to another thirty days "as a warning to others who contemplated escape." The admonition failed. Instead, between June and July, another sixteen women escaped the confines of the hospital.

The hospital's managers responded by increasing their surveillance. This proved effective because the total number of women escaping declined down to the single digits in the 1920s. In retrospect, Cosgrove argued that the inmates required constant supervision "because of their mentality."[75] Social worker Helen M. Kemp believed that the drop resulted from the hospital's personnel exercising "a greater watchfulness and more resourcefulness in preventing escapes and in maintaining discipline without the aid of police."[76] Yet the fear that women desired to escape remained a recurring concern.

While the managers of Los Feliz Hospital attributed the decline in escapees to their actions within the facility itself, they also noted that changes in criminal procedure affected inmates' outlooks. According to Bettin, the women exhibited "a great deal of unrest and anxiety" because the city quarantined them before they were convicted of any crime.[77] As the health department pursued a more vigorous policy because of World War I, the women who became the court's subjects turned to them for relief. Working-class women found that requesting habeas corpus, a legal order requiring officials to bring the petitioner before the court to determine the legality of her detention, was an effective means for them to challenge public health actions. From 1917 to 1918, habeas corpus had been used in a variety of criminal cases in Los Angeles, ranging from murder, fraud, and custody disputes to driving a bus without a license.[78] In at least two instances, the cases involved releasing minors from the Preston

School of Industry, a juvenile detention center.[79] According to historian David J. Pivar, the Chamberlain-Kahn Act suspended women's rights to sue for habeas corpus if they were arrested for violating health laws. The application of this law, however, was contested.[80] Moreover, the women who sued in Los Angeles had been arrested for violating municipal anti-vice ordinances, not health codes or federal law. At first, women filed their petitions with the municipal courts, and they sometimes won. Once they started consistently losing in the city's judicial system, however, they began to appeal their cases to the California Appellate Court. The evidence delineates a process by which local officials sought to define dangerous behaviors.

The first case mentioned by health officials in their annual reports was heard by the municipal courts in 1918 and involved two African American women.[81] The police arrested the two women on drug charges, and the health department quarantined them because, according to Jeancon, they were "known prostitutes." Jeancon ordered an examination but the women refused. Instead, they filed a writ of habeas corpus. The court ruled in the petitioners' favor, arguing that only in charges "involving moral turpitude" could the health department quarantine. Although the health department lost this first case, Jeancon believed that the court legitimized the city's power and she contended that "women now rarely refuse[d] examination and a great many, on learning of their condition, volunteer to go to Los Feliz Hospital for treatment" because of these decisions. Despite Jeancon's assertion, the legitimacy of public policy regarding venereal disease and the ability of the health department to translate that policy into reality remained arguable.

In petitioning for a writ of habeas corpus, women exposed officials' lack of certainty regarding enforcement of their public health policies. Local representatives met with state officials to strategize a response as well as to clarify points of issue. In June 1918, Kemper B. Campbell, state attorney for the state board of health, Los Angeles superior court justice Willis, the city health commissioner L. M. Powers, and three other prominent local physicians met at the California Club for an informal conference.[82] Willis's recent release of two women from county jail who had petitioned for a writ of habeas corpus provoked the discussion. Willis explained that he granted their freedom because the county had not provided a place for quarantine.

Originally the city had agreed to take in county cases based on the understanding that the county would contribute to the expenses of running Los Feliz. After one year, however, the county had not allocated any funds. The city health department declared its "embarrassment" in having to take care of county needs and, citing tight finances, stopped accepting county cases.

Conscious of its borders, the city argued that taxpayers of the county should create their own hospital for patients with venereal disease.

Willis affirmed the powers of public health officials at the same time that he found for the petitioners. He reminded those present that he had consistently denied writs at the city level. At the end of the conference, Willis agreed to speak with the two other superior court judges who he felt would be likely to hear similar cases. He promised that he would ask his colleagues to join him in a united petition to the county board of supervisors requesting the creation of appropriate accommodations. In the meantime, Willis offered a way around the problem. He suggested that the county transfer patients to the county hospital.

Besides strategizing at this June meeting, Powers raised questions about the extent of power given to local authorities. Powers asked Campbell whether the city had the right to draw blood for the Wassermann test over the objections of the suspect. Campbell believed that the city would be within its rights, yet he recommended against it because of public objections. Instead, he proposed holding suspects in confinement until they acquiesced.[83] Powers's question might not have been a hypothetical one. At the time of this meeting, the "imbibing [but] respectable woman" was three months into her act of civil disobedience. While public health officials sorted out the implementation of state and federal regulations at the municipal level, women moved beyond the local courts in their attempts to resist such laws. Habeas corpus petitions began to reach the Court of Appeals for the first time in late 1918.

On Armistice Day, November 11, 1918, Los Angeles police officer C. F. Johnson took Grace Johnston into custody from 4150 Third Avenue.[84] Apparently, Johnston's mother had informed police that her daughter was carrying on "adulterous relations with one Thomas Harry Johnston." Grace Johnston contested this characterization and argued that she was removed from her home where she had been "surrounded by her own friends and relatives." Furthermore, while claiming to be a policeman, Officer C. F. Johnson had not produced a warrant for her arrest. Once in the city jail, Grace Johnston submitted to an examination by Mona Bettin, who determined that she had a case of infectious gonorrhea. The next day, still without being brought before a judge, Johnston found herself transferred to Los Feliz. There she remained and underwent treatments for gonorrhea for about two weeks, until she sued for habeas corpus. The local Superior Court released her on bail until a hearing could be held. At this hearing, Johnston argued that she had never been afflicted with gonorrhea, producing affidavits from "two reputable physicians" to prove her innocence. She attempted to fight science with science.[85] But she lost her petition at that hearing on February 8, 1919, and was remanded to Los Feliz, where she "steadfastly refused . . . to permit any examination of her person."

Johnston appealed to the California Appellate Court. Johnston's lawyer, Paul W. Schenck, a defense attorney in Los Angeles, based her petition on the tenet that no person can be deprived of life, liberty, or property without due process of law.[86] If the lower court's interpretation of the state act stood, he argued, it would make the law "the most revolutionary act as was ever passed by any legislature since the foundation of this government." Furthermore, Schenck argued that the issue went deeper than merely wrongful imprisonment. This law, he contended, carried significant social ramifications for the women whose lives it affected because any "lowly uneducated policeman on the beat . . . may publicly and officially degrade, humiliate and forever blight the lives of these poor victims, by carrying them from the bosom of their families and incarcerating them in a bastille indefinitely." In addition, Schenck stressed that the damage was greater than mere disgrace because it was actually a physical violation because the government could "not only invade the security and sacredness of their person but also inject them with such serums and fluids as they may see fit."

The counsel for the city of Los Angeles accused Schenck of making inflammatory and deceitful remarks. As a friend to city's counsel, Campbell argued that this public health policy had "nothing to do with morals" and that Johnston remained in quarantine because of the infectious state within which she existed. Although Johnston had aroused the city's suspicion for allegedly being a "lewd and dissolute person," a crime she was not actually charged with until she sued, Campbell maintained that detention was "a health measure and not a penal procedure." Relying on the oral testimony of Mona Bettin, the court found in favor of the city. But they made a qualification. The appellate court stated that it had originally issued the writ based on the belief that Johnston had not been afflicted and, in fact, conceded that if that had been proven in court they would have released her. Scientific proof of infection, thus, became essential for the state to exercise its powers.

On August 24, 1919, a special police squad known as the "Purity Squad" (an undercover unit that enjoyed a long and contentious history in the city's police department) showed up at a lodging house at 106 W. Tenth Street at one o'clock in the morning and arrested Frank Dillon, Ethel Adams, Florence Milstead, Jessie Eades, and Mary Smith for violating City Ordinance 25640, or "The Rooming-House Ordinance."[87] This was passed as part of a larger movement in Los Angeles to suppress vice in its various forms but was not specifically a public health reform. Since the amendment of state law in 1917 that made city officials representatives of the state, the city health department had been examining all persons charged in violation. Based on these investigations, the city estimated that about 90 percent of the women arrested for breaking this law had proven infectious. World War I was over, but the health department used this statistic to justify the continuation of its policy.

The litigants quickly sued for habeas corpus. The court granted them a hearing and allowed the petitioners to be released on bail until that time. At this point, no examinations had taken place. Dillon was freed on $250 bail while each of the women had to produce only $25 (a disparity that suggests Dillon was their pimp). On the day of the hearing, a confusing court drama unfolded. Only Dillon and Adams presented themselves before the court. Milstead, Eades, and Smith failed to appear. According to their lawyer, all of them had left for San Francisco. The superior court judge decided to remand Dillon and Adams to jail. Before they could be removed from the courtroom, however, their lawyers managed to serve an appended writ upon the chief of police that prevented him from taking them into custody.

The petitioners' lawyers appealed the case to the appellate court. The defendants cited the Magna Carta, the Declaration of Rights, and the Declaration of Independence, but they actually won their case because the city could not prove that any of them were afflicted with venereal disease. "In fact, [the court wrote, the rooming-house ordinance] would seem to exclude persons committing illicit sexual acts at their established place of abode, regardless of the character of such persons." The court asked whether "the health department may reasonably assume, without any pervious knowledge, information, or report as to the individual concerned, that every person arrested by officers and booked at the city jail as having violated the "Rooming-House Ordinance" is reasonably likely to be afflicted with a quarantinable venereal disease." Public health reformers would have said yes, but the court's answer was no. The court continued to ask the health department to be more specific in its arguments about who was "reasonably" suspect.

On April 9, 1921, an undercover cop named Terrill Hahn took a walk down New High Street at 10:30 at night.[88] There he encountered Frank Perry standing on the sidewalk and asked him if he knew "where he could get a girl." Perry kindly escorted him to house number 643 and knocked on the door. Mrs. A. Arata answered. After Perry and Arata exchanged a few words in Spanish, she "invited" Hahn inside, where they settled on a price of two dollars. Hahn handed her a five-dollar bill that she put in a vase and gave him change. Already "scantily clad," Arata lay down on the bed. A moment later, two police officers "kicked in the door" and arrested her for prostitution.

As was the standard practice, a woman physician working for the health department attempted to examine Arata for venereal disease in the jail; she refused. At the arraignment two days later, she pleaded not guilty and the judge set bail at $50. Arata paid but to her surprise this did not secure her release. The health department forbade her discharge until she submitted to an examination. Using Paul Schenk, Johnston's former attorney, Arata responded by petitioning the California Court of Appeals for a writ of habeas corpus. She argued that she never had venereal disease and that she was not a prostitute. Health officials countered that the circumstances surrounding her arrest suggested that Arata was a prostitute and therefore probably infected.

The Court of Appeals found in favor of Arata and she was freed. The court decided that, at the time of the arrest, no act of prostitution had actually been performed. Although city health officials and the police had charged her with prostitution, they had offered no proof. While siding with Arata, the court outlined a specific legal test for health authorities to follow in the future. Officials needed to demonstrate a suspect's previous exposure to venereal disease. Prostitutes, the court declared, could be considered as a "class" who it was reasonable to believe had been exposed to venereal disease. The court required health authorities to prove that the suspect belonged to this "class." This burden of proof, the court suggested, could be met by providing evidence of prior convictions for this type of crime.

A few weeks later, Betty Dayton tested these standards.[89] On April 28, 1921, between 10:30 and 11 P.M., H. W. Scott, a clerk of the police court, and Frank P. Mohler went to the New Broadway Hotel. There Scott spoke with taxi driver E. A. Conway, asking him "if he knew where there was a live 'joint' and declared that 'this is the deadest town I have been into for a long time. I thought there were some wild women here.'" Conway allegedly replied, "What do you mean a dead town? I will take you to the livest place in Los Angeles." So Conway drove Scott and Mohler to the corner of Third and Rampart. He left them in the car while he went up to Number 267 South Rampart Street and spoke with its female African American residents who came to the door wearing kimonos. At Scott's request, Conway asked how much it would be to stay. The women allegedly stated $10 for once or $20 for the entire night. Scott then bought a round of drinks, for which he paid in marked bills. He knew he needed to contact the sergeant as well as delay the proceedings. Under the pretense of calling another friend to join them, Scott suggested that they all ride in the taxi to a place where he could telephone. Stating that they expected payment for accompanying Scott, Valentine Berryman and Jean Stetson changed out of their kimonos. Scott phoned the sergeant and then they returned to the brothel. Shortly upon returning, the police arrived and arrested everyone in the house, including another woman, Marie Baldwin, who had not been a part of the party.

The police charged all of these women with being "idle, lewd, and dissolute person[s]." The police docket transcript also reveals that the judge wanted Dayton to admit she was running a brothel, which she finally did. She maintained, however, that she did not engage in acts of prostitution. According to her writ, Dayton, upon the advice of counsel, pleaded guilty and was sentenced to a $150 fine or 150 days in jail for "keeping a disorderly house" and for selling liquor. Dayton chose to pay the fines but found herself still subject to quarantine. In her complaint she argued that she had never been afflicted with a venereal disease and that the health department had no reason to suspect her because at the time of the arrest she had not engaged in an act of intercourse.

The court decided that it was "not essential that the particular acts indulged in such houses be expressly shown." Instead, it was enough that "all of the surroundings, as the evidence illustrated them [referring to the police docket transcript], the actions, conduct, and demeanor of the persons occupying the place in the aggregate establish . . . quite clearly and beyond a probability . . . that the house was a house of ill fame and that the inmates belonged to the class mentioned." The court viewed any engagement in the sex trade as unhealthy enough to be defined as a threat to society. After *in re Dayton*, women only sporadically appealed their cases to the state and they were consistently denied.[90]

The story ended in an interesting coda. The decision was handed down May 13, 1921, and approximately a week later some of the defendants took matters into their own hands. Stetson, Baldwin, Berryman, and five other women "escaped from the first floor of the hospital by breaking a small padlock from one of the windows. . . . Jumping to the ground, the woman grabbed a long plank and placed it against the woven wire fence. Then they ran up this gang plank and jumped to the Los Feliz Road and freedom."[91]

What happened to Los Feliz? Although the city put serious financial resources into the hospital during World War I, including purchasing a stove, water heater, 500-gallon water-storage tank, and 2000-gallon oil tank, the city did not purchase any major equipment or make any major structural improvements in the 1920s. Without sustained support for its physical infrastructure, the hospital slowly disintegrated. Citing broken windows, heaters, a leaky roof, worn floors, and rotting doors, a grand jury condemned the facility in 1924.[92] Four years later, the city council's health committee determined that the building's disrepair had become even more hazardous. For instance, it found that "the wood in the treatment tables has so badly rotted that the tables are no longer safe." The committee estimated that it would cost the city almost a thousand dollars to make the necessary repairs.[93] Neither report, however, stopped the city from using the facilities up until its closure on January 9, 1932, when the city just could not afford it anymore. Although closed, it was not forgotten. As early as 1934, the city health officer, George Parrish, made overtures to reopen the hospital.[94] In September 1941, Minnie Barton, a parole officer of the city police department, spoke to the Woman's City Club about the accomplishments of their forerunners. She argued that "the things you have worked so far for have gone, including those two badly needed institutions, the Woman's Court and the Los Feliz Hospital." She asked for women to reopen the facility and to pressure the city to do more for women in need.[95] Her call, apparently, went unheeded.

During the era of World War I, female reformers' assumptions about dangerous behaviors helped form public health measures in Los Angeles. While reformers and public health officials began their efforts prior to the Great War, this event proved pivotal for the implementation of social hygienists' ambitions to conquer vice and of health officials' desire to create an extensive venereal-disease program. California expanded the legislative powers of local health departments under federal pressure to maintain a healthy combat force. The wartime boom also generated the funds with which health departments could execute their plans. In addition, the draft publicized the prevalence of venereal disease, allowing for a more public discussion.

In exploring the relationship between technologies of treatment and public health policies, the evidence for Los Angeles suggests that changes in medical knowledge did not automatically modify policy. Instead policies were tempered by social contexts. In this case, although World War I had a major impact on public health campaigns against venereal disease, it also indicates that these changes were not without limitation or complexity. For instance, the treatment available for syphilis was greatly impacted by the war because of the increased access to Salvarsan. Yet, the treatment for gonorrhea remained much the same as before the war.

While the city health officials' powers were expanded because of the war, this expansion did not go unchallenged. Health officials were confronted with the unexpected; the accused sometimes successfully challenged definitions of what behaviors could lead the health department to "reasonably" suspect someone as a venereal disease carrier. The courts restricted the application of the anti-vice ordinances that had been conceived by reformers a decade earlier. At the same time, the court expanded the state's power over women's bodies in the criminal justice system. Thus, the breadth of female reformers' vision of public health became increasingly limited in the hands of officials.

Conclusion

Current debates over how to reform health insurance indicate that many people remain uncommitted to intensifying government's role in promoting the public's health, even for the most vulnerable in our society. These disputes stand in contrast to what reformers achieved in Los Angeles during the early twentieth century. In 1889, the Los Angeles city health department consisted of a single health officer whose expense account amounted to $1,200 for the entire year. By 1932, the department was divided into fifteen special divisions and its expenditures totaled over $700,000. Health officials spent much of this money on programs that brought medical care into working people's homes even when confronted by the financial woes of the 1930s.

The Great Depression created new pressures on the city government to provide more health services with less money. As the chief health officer at the time, C. W. Decker, commented: "Economic conditions ha[d] laid unusual burdens upon Public Health" and there had been a "drastic curtailment" of the budget."[1] Decker saved money by mimeographing the annual report instead of sending it to the printing press. The fiscal crisis put two health programs created by female reformers in peril: the city's maternity service and Los Feliz Hospital. The housing and nursing divisions, however, still received significant funds. Combined, the two divisions composed 39 percent of the health department's overall operating expenses in 1932.[2] These programs became the primary means by which the city protected the public's health during this precarious time. The New Deal changed people's orientation and expectations of the federal government and its relationship to state and local municipalities, but a basic assumption about government's capacity to provide health services had already been laid into place. In Los Angeles, women were directly responsible for expanding the breadth of the city's public health infrastructure prior to this calamitous event.

Because public health did not reach maturity as a distinct profession until the 1930s, it offered a forum for women with disparate interests but a common concern for the public's health to engage in reform. They concocted systemic solutions to coping with life in a modern city. Cityscape was sometimes a backdrop but more often it was an actor in debates over public health policy. Despite booster rhetoric, conditions of poverty existed. Female reformers crafted programs for public health nursing, housing renovation, birthing services, and venereal disease treatment to transform unhealthy environments. In the case of milk reform, reformers attempted to offset their anxieties about the separation between consumers and their food sources.

These issues were not unique to Los Angeles. Across the nation, reformers identified similar problems: living conditions, medical care, and food safety. Networks explain this consistency of perspective across different urban geographies. Renowned figures such as Jane Addams, James B. Reynolds, Florence Kelley, Graham Taylor, and Jacob Riis who visited Los Angeles did so as part of a larger lecture circuit. These eminent reformers crisscrossed the United States providing a paradigm for articulating health hazards. Their trips to Los Angeles inspired women to reexamine their assumptions about local conditions and to engage in advocacy. Yet the dominant discourse of reform they presented for conceptualizing public health problems did not exactly match the city's particular residential architecture, dynamics of immigration, food distribution system, and shape of city politics. Local circumstances prompted reformers in Los Angeles to adopt a unique strategy: reformulate the city's public health infrastructure by modifying city government.

Los Angeles women expanded the city health department's focus from reaction to prevention. They did this by creating programs for the distribution of health services for the city to adopt. Based on their faith in the capacity of government to effect social change, the women of the Los Angeles College Settlement Association took the lead in building a relationship with the city's health administrators. They derived their power from sympathy and science. Working in a period wherein it was unclear what responsibility lay with the private or public sector, their invention of a semimunicipal program for public health nursing provided precedence for an active government. Women's clubs and social hygienists built upon the settlement's experience to further increase the scope of the health department's administration. Through these combined actions reformers brought municipal health services into people's homes and neighborhoods. In doing so, they changed perceptions about the city.

Women could do this because they worked within a gray area. They facilitated connections between residents and their city government although they did not act as official representatives. Nonetheless, throughout all of these chapters of transformation in the city's history, reformers' records betray their lack of control over the public's consumption of their services. Challenges came in the form of overt resistance and more subtle acts of stubbornness. They faced opposition from the general public, other reformers, politicians, patients, and private physicians. Conflict depended upon the disease in question, time, and place. In the case of milk reform, women of similar social standing but different philosophical outlooks battled one another over what was in the best interests of their families. In the case of venereal disease treatment, reformers had to modify the length of treatment in order to stem conflict within Los Feliz Hospital. Within homes, patients and their families picked elements of these programs in accordance with their own needs and beliefs about how to promote health, and reformers needed to negotiate with them if they wanted to be effective. In the end, reformers made compromises to achieve their goals.

Female reformers' relationship with city officials was complex. At various moments the chief health officer, Luther Milton Powers, supported their interests and at other times he appears to have receded into the background. His ambiguous stance presumably proved politic for retaining his position from 1897 until his death in 1924. In contrast, LACSA's relationship with the city's public health policy makers, the board of health, was a different matter. When there was official opposition to its programs, it typically came from this panel of four elite physicians who owed their appointment to the city council (the mayor served as the fifth member). At various moments, such as responding to an outbreak of measles in 1910, these physicians found women's assertion of authority over medical matters a threat to their power. Yet, it does not appear that they objected in theory to increasing the breadth of the health department. Arguments about the loss of patients to public services had not yet become a pressing issue for this local medical community.

As European scientists offered new theories on the origin of disease that traced specific illnesses to particular microscopic living organisms, reformers were equipped with new arguments to legitimize their work. In the case of syphilis, Ehrlich's discovery of Salvarsan aided public health measures. In the case of milk, scientific debates derailed reformers' efforts. Women's greatest public policy success came when they pursued areas of reform that focused on the application of sanitary practices instead of the science behind it. They also exerted greater control over policy when the public perceived the area to be a subject of infant and maternal health. Beliefs about gender roles, hence, simultaneously served as a source of power and as a limitation.

While the responses of patients pushed female reformers to adjust their programs, these policy makers were also informed by their own prejudices. Over time, stereotypes changed. For instance, reformers reimagined Mexicans from being pleasantly pliable to dangerously intractable. Still, they always assumed that Russians, Italians, Slovaks, and Mexicans were culpable for disease transmission. The only question for reformers was whether these residents were cognizant of their role. Anxieties about assimilation and health practices converged. However, where immigrants adopted modern medicine, these concerns were mitigated. Italian and Japanese midwives continued to practice because their diplomas abrogated anxieties about their ethnicities.

Protests over the closure of programs for venereal disease and maternity services convey women's sense of ownership over these programs even when they ceased to run their day-to-day activities. Reformers did not object to the professionalization of the health department because at first women retained a voice in forming public policy by sitting on the commissions that oversaw the nursing, housing, and venereal disease programs. The adoption of a new city charter, which was promoted as the vanguard of progressive political reform by its supporters, eliminated these structures in 1924. The new charter returned the power over public health policy to an appointive citizen board of five members whose appointments were made by the mayor. This new board of health was controlled by medical men and businessmen. Excluded from these positions, women lost control over their programs. But this is not a story of lamentation. Female reformers changed the city's orientation and societal expectations about public health services. They not only introduced the idea of government responsibility for promoting health but created a model. The city was not an imagined community to them but a real one, where everyone's health interests were interlinked and still are.

Access to affordable health care remains a pressing issue. While the specific dynamics have changed, broad universal questions remain about the role of government-assisted public health measures for the most vulnerable populations. Current debates ask who is better at taking the initiative to protect the public's health: volunteer organizations or the state? Arguments over subsidizing faith-based associations that provide drug rehabilitation and school vouchers are just two examples of the struggles to determine the proper distribution of public resources. Providing public funds to private groups to experiment with and maintain health-related programs calls into question the nature of government's role. In the way in which these discussions are framed, private and public administrations are depicted as being inherently in conflict. Yet, Los Angeles women in the early twentieth century did not look at expanding the role of volunteer or government agencies as exclusive solutions. Their model offers an alternative approach for thinking about the broad array of actors who can work in collaboration to find answers to critical public health matters.

Abbreviations

HDAR	Annual Report of the Health Department of the City of Los Angeles
HDMR	Monthly Report of the Health Department of the City of Los Angeles
HCR	Report of the Housing Commission of the City of Los Angeles
IDNR	Report of Instructive District Nursing for the City of Los Angeles Under the Supervision of the College Settlement
KPE Collection	Katherine Philips Edson Papers
LACA	Los Angeles City Archives, Erwin C. Piper Technical Center
LC	Library of Congress
NYPL	New York Public Library

Notes

Introduction

1. *Report of Instructive District Nursing for the City of Los Angeles under the Supervision of the College Settlement* (1908–1910): 9–10 (hereafter *IDNR*).
2. Charles E. Rosenberg, *The Care of Strangers: The Rise of America's Hospital System* (Baltimore: Johns Hopkins University Press, 1987).
3. Martin Melosi, *The Sanitary City: Urban Infrastructure in America from Colonial Times to the Present* (Baltimore: Johns Hopkins University Press, 2000); Eric H. Monkkonen, *America Becomes Urban: The Development of U.S. Cities and Towns, 1780–1980* (Berkeley: University of California Press, 1990), 93–95; Charles E. Rosenberg, *The Cholera Years: The United States in 1832, 1849, and 1866* (Chicago: University of Chicago Press, 1962).
4. Nancy Tomes, *The Gospel of Germs: Men, Women, and the Microbe in American Life* (Cambridge, Mass.: Harvard University Press, 1998).
5. Theda Skocpol, *Protecting Soldiers and Mothers: The Political Origins of Social Policy in the United States* (Cambridge, Mass.: Belknap Press of Harvard University Press, 1992), 43.
6. By way of example, see John Duffy, *The Sanitarians: A History of American Public Health* (Urbana: University of Illinois Press, 1990); Evelynn Maxine Hammonds, *Childhood's Deadly Scourge: The Campaign to Control Diphtheria in New York City, 1890–1930* (Baltimore: Johns Hopkins University Press, 1999); Judith Walzer Leavitt, *The Healthiest City: Milwaukee and the Politics of Health Reform* (Madison: University of Wisconsin Press, 1982); Howard Markel, *Quarantine!: East European Jewish Immigrants and the New York City Epidemics of 1892* (Baltimore: Johns Hopkins University Press, 1997).
7. See Linda Gordon, *Pitied but Not Entitled: Single Mothers and the History of Welfare* (New York: Free Press, 1994), and Skocpol, *Protecting Soldiers*.
8. See Janis Appier, *The Sexual Politics of Law Enforcement and the LAPD* (Philadelphia: Temple University Press, 1998); Anastasia J. Christman, "The Best Laid Plans: Women's Clubs and City Planning in Los Angeles, 1890–1930" (Ph.D. diss., UCLA, 2000); Sarah Deutsch, *Women and the City: Gender, Space, and Power in Boston, 1870–940* (New York: Oxford University Press, 2000); Maureen A. Flanagan, *Seeing with Their Hearts: Chicago Women and the Vision of the Good City, 1871–1933* (Princeton, N.J.: Princeton University Press, 2002); Estelle Freedman, *Maternal Justice: Miriam Van Waters and the Female Reform Tradition* (Chicago: University of Chicago Press, 1996); Gayle Gullet, *Becoming Citizens: The Emergence and Development of the California Women's Movement, 1880–1911* (Urbana: University of Illinois Press, 2000); Mary Odem, *Delinquent Daughters: Protecting Adolescent Female Sexuality in the United States, 1885–1920* (Chapel Hill: University of North Carolina Press, 1995); Daphne Spain, *How Women Saved the City* (Minneapolis: University of Minnesota Press, 2000).
9. See Lynne Curry, *Modern Mothers in the Heartland: Gender, Health, and Progress in Illinois, 1900–1930* (Columbus: Ohio State University Press, 1999); Robyn Muncy, *Creating a Female Dominion in American Reform, 1890–1935* (New York: Oxford

University Press, 1994); Jacqueline H. Wolf, *Don't Kill Your Baby: Public Health and the Decline of Breastfeeding in the Nineteenth and Twentieth Centuries* (Columbus: Ohio State University Press, 2001).

10. Sherry Jeanne Katz, "Dual Commitments: Feminism, Socialism, and Women's Political Activism in California, 1890–1920" (Ph.D. diss., UCLA, 1991), 48. Regarding Edward Bellamy, see Arthur Morgan, *Edward Bellamy* (New York: Columbia University Press, 1944); John L. Thomas, *Alternative America: Henry George, Edward Bellamy, Henry Demarest Lloyd and the Adversary Tradition* (Cambridge, Mass.: Belknap Press of Harvard University Press, 1983).

11. Gerald Woods argues that Southern Californians' penchant for probity stemmed from their ethnicity and religion. See Gerald Woods, "A Penchant for Probity: California Progressives and the Disreputable Pleasures," in *California Progressivism Revisited*, ed. William Deverell and Tom Sitton (Berkeley: University of California Press, 1994), 109.

12. *Annual Report of the Health Department of the City of Los Angeles* (1904), 17 (hereafter *HDAR*).

13. "Land of Sunshine" is a reference to the title of a journal produced by the infamous Charles Fletcher Lummis. The literature on Los Angeles boosterism is vast. A few that have informed my interpretation are Mike Davis, *City of Quartz: Excavating the Future in Los Angeles* (London: Verso, 1990); William Deverell, *Whitewashed Adobe: The Rise of Los Angeles and the Remaking of Its Mexican Past* (Berkeley: University of California Press, 2004); Lee M. A. Simpson, *Selling the City: Gender, Class, and the California Growth Machine, 1880–1940* (Stanford, Calif.: Stanford University Press, 2004); Kevin Starr, *Material Dreams: Southern California through the 1920s* (New York: Oxford University Press, 1991).

14. See Susan Craddock, *City of Plagues: Disease, Poverty, and Deviance in San Francisco* (Minneapolis: University of Minnesota Press, 2000); Deverell, *Whitewashed Adobe*, chapter 5; Amy Fairchild, *Science at the Borders: Immigrant Medical Inspection and the Shaping of the Modern Industrial Labor Force* (Baltimore: Johns Hopkins University Press, 2003); Alan M. Kraut, *Silent Travelers: Germs, Genes, and the Immigrant Menace* (Baltimore: Johns Hopkins University Press, 1995); Natalia Molina, *Fit to Be Citizens?: Public Health and Race in Los Angeles, 1879–1939* (Berkeley: University of California Press, 2006); Nayan Shah, *Contagious Divides: Epidemics and Race in San Francisco's Chinatown* (Berkeley: University of California Press, 2001).

15. See Emily Abel, "From Exclusion to Expulsion: Mexicans and Tuberculosis Control in Los Angeles, 1914–1940," *Bulletin of the History of Medicine* 77.4 (2003): 823–884; Emily Abel, *Tuberculosis and the Politics of Exclusion: A History of Public Health and Migration in Los Angeles* (New Brunswick, N.J.: Rutgers University Press, 2007).

16. Robert M. Fogelson, *Fragmented Metropolis: Los Angeles, 1850–1930*, (Cambridge, Mass.: Harvard University Press, 1968), chapter 4; George Sanchez, *Becoming Mexican American: Ethnicity, Culture and Identity in Chicano Los Angeles, 1900–1945* (New York: Oxford University Press, 1993), chapter 3.

17. On women's clubs as spaces for the development of a political and social identity, see Karen Blair, *The Clubwoman as Feminist: True Womanhood Redefined, 1868–1914* (New York: Holmes and Meier, 1980); Flanagan, *Seeing with Their Hearts*; Estelle Freedman, "Separatism as Strategy: Female Institution Building and American Feminism, 1870–1930," *Feminist Studies* 5 (Fall 1979): 512–529; Muncy,

Creating a Female Dominion; Anne Firor Scott, *Natural Allies: Women's Associations in American History* (Urbana: University of Illinois Press, 1991); Kathryn Kish Sklar, "Hull House in the 1890s: A Community of Female Reformers," *Signs* 10, no. 4 (Summer 1985): 658–677. On the history of the Friday Morning Club, see Judith Raftery, "Los Angeles Clubwomen and Progressive Reform," in *California Progressivism Revisited*, ed. William Deverell and Tom Sitton (Berkeley: University of California Press, 1994), 147–153.

18. Programs for November 1893, April 1894, and November 1894, Box 83, Folder 11, Severance Collection, Huntington Library.
19. "Friday Morning Club," *Los Angeles Herald*, February 3, 1894. Regarding the politicization of women's consumerism, see Rebecca Edwards, *Angels in the Machinery: Gender in American Party Politics from the Civil War to the Progressive Era* (New York: Oxford University Press, 1997).
20. For historical perspectives on Jane Addams and Hull House, see Victoria Bissell Brown, *The Education of Jane Addams* (Philadelphia: University of Pennsylvania Press, 2004); Allen F. Davis, *American Heroine: The Life and Legend of Jane Addams* (New York: Oxford University Press, 1973); Jean Bethke Elshtain, *Jane Addams and the Dream of American Democracy* (New York: Basic Books, 2002). James Bronson Reynolds is best known for his appointment by President Theodore Roosevelt to investigate the meatpacking industry after the publication of *The Jungle*. See Allen F. Davis, *Spearheads for Reform: The Social Settlements and the Progressive Movement, 1890–1914* (New York: Oxford University Press, 1967), 28; *The National Cyclopedia of American Biography*, vols. 10:235 and 33:182.
21. "Friday Morning Club," *Los Angeles Herald*, February 3, 1894; "Friday Morning Club," *Los Angeles Express*, February 3, 1894; Editorial, "Our Ethical Condition," *Los Angeles Express*, February 3, 1894.
22. I have been unable to unearth any archival evidence that would provide an exact birth and death date for LACSA. The only document that indicates its official establishment says "February 1894." See *The First Report of the Los Angeles Settlements Association at Casa de Castelar* (Los Angeles: B. R. Baumgardt, 1897), 4. See also Michael E. Engh, "Mary J. Workman: The Catholic Conscience of Los Angeles," *California History*, Spring 1993, 7. Regarding the Collegiate Alumni Association of Los Angeles, see "In Social Spheres: Collegiate Alumnae Reception," *Los Angeles Times*, May 16, 1894; "In Social Spheres: A Luncheon," *Los Angeles Times*, January 14, 1896; "In Social Spheres: The Wellesley Club," *Los Angeles Times*, July 16, 1896; and "Society," *Los Angeles Times*, January 27, 1897.
23. Unfortunately no roster from the FMC exists to compare its membership with that of the Collegiate Alumni Association of Los Angeles for February 1894.
24. "Alumnae Reception," *Los Angeles Times*, January 20, 1894.
25. Daniel T. Rodgers, *Atlantic Crossings: Social Politics in the Progressive Era* (Cambridge, Mass.: Belknap Press of Harvard University Press, 1998).
26. Historiographical debates on settlement houses often vacillate between describing them as venues for vanguard social activism and feminist empowerment or the means for maintaining systems of racial and economic oppression. But either characterization, as historian Ruth Crocker has argued, moves away from the historical experience of the residents who either staffed or received services from these types of institutions. Instead, settlements were sites of complex interaction. See Ruth Crocker, *Social Work and Social Order: The Settlement Movement in Two Industrial Cities, 1889–1930* (Urbana: University of Illinois Press, 1992), 8–9.

27. Congregationalists founded the Bethlehem Institute in 1892. Mary J. Workman established the Brownson House as a Catholic institution in 1904. Episcopalians created the Neighborhood House in 1910. The same year, the Council of Jewish Women formed the Stinson Memorial Industrial School. See Robert A. Woods, *Handbook of Settlements* (New York: Charities Publication Committee, 1911).

28. See Stanley K. Schultz, *Constructing Urban Culture: American Cities and City Planning, 1800–1920* (Philadelphia: Temple University Press, 1989).

29. Historians have noted at least two other instances of women using science and sympathy. See Robert D. Johnston, *The Radical Middle Class: Populist Democracy and the Question of Capitalism in Progressive Era Portland, Oregon* (Princeton, N.J.: Princeton University Press, 2006); Howard L. Platt, "Jane Addams and the Ward Boss Revisited: Class, Politics, and Public Health in Chicago, 1890–1930," *Environmental History* 5 (April 2000): 194–222.

30. Margaret Humphreys, *Malaria: Poverty, Race, and Public Health in the United States* (Baltimore: Johns Hopkins University Press, 2001), 5.

Chapter 1: Paid for by the Public Purse

1. For consistency I will use the term "public health nursing" throughout this chapter even though the term did not come into vogue until the National Organization of Public Health Nursing (NOPHN) was formed in 1912. See Karen Buhler-Wilkerson, *False Dawn: The Rise and Decline of Public Health Nursing, 1900–1930* (New York: Garland, 1989), 137–138.

2. City Archives Petitions No. 650 (1897), Los Angeles City Archives, Erwin C. Piper Technical Center (hereafter LACA).

3. Board of Health Minutes, May 15, 1895, LACA. See also Engh, "Mary Julia Workman," 7.

4. Katz, "Socialist Women and Progressive Reform," in *California Progressivism Revisited*, ed. Deverell and Sitton, 117–143.

5. Mary K. Sedgwick, "Instructive District Nursing," *Forum* 22 (1896): 300; Yssabella Waters, *Visiting Nursing in the United States* (New York: Charities Publication Committee, 1909), 315–364.

6. City Council Minutes, vol. 51, page 221 (1897), LACA. Archival research has not yielded any additional information about Toll's motivation.

7. Karen Buhler-Wilkerson's interpretive work on home care provides the most comprehensive analysis of public health nursing as a movement. She looks at public health nursing, however, from the perspective of the NOPHN and from eastern and southern associations. Although aspects of Los Angeles's story sound similar to Buhler-Wilkerson's findings, I believe that my research demonstrates that the public funding of Los Angeles's program and differences in management requires a revision of our understanding of this history. See Karen Buhler-Wilkerson, *No Place Like Home: A History of Nursing and Home Care in the United States* (Baltimore: Johns Hopkins University Press, 2001). See also Barbara Melosh, *"The Physician's Hand": Work Culture and Conflict in American Nursing* (Philadelphia: Temple University Press, 1982), chapter 4; Susan Reverby, *Ordered to Care: The Dilemma of American Nursing, 1850–1945* (New York: Cambridge University Press, 1987), 109–110.

8. Annie M. Brainard, *The Evolution of Public Health Nursing* (Philadelphia: W. B. Saunders, 1922), 102–118; Waters, *Visiting Nursing in the United States*, 13; Buhler-Wilkerson, *No Place Like Home*, 18–22; Buhler-Wilkerson, *False Dawn*, 6–7; Eleanor F. Rathbone, *William Rathbone: A Memoir* (London: Macmillan, 1905), 155–186.

9. Waters, *Visiting Nursing*, 315–364.
10. *IDNR* (1898–1907), 7. See also the Los Angeles Settlement Association, *The College Settlement, Los Angeles, California* (Los Angeles, 1905), 10.
11. Kathryn Kish Sklar, "Who Funded Hull Huse?" in *Lady Bountiful Revisited: Women, Philanthropy, and Power*, ed Kathleen D. McCarthy (New Brunswick: N.J.: Rutgers University Press, 1990), 95–115. See also Buhler-Wilkerson, *No Place Like Home*, chapter 1.
12. *First Report of the Los Angeles Settlements Association at Casa de Castelar* (Los Angeles: B. R. Baumgardt, 1897), 22 and 30.
13. *IDNR* (1898–1907), 7. See also the Los Angeles Settlement Association, *The College Settlement*, 10.
14. Los Angeles Board of Health Minutes, February 23, 1897, and March 9, 1897, LACA; City Council Minutes vol. 50, pages 590–593 (1897), LACA; City Council Minutes vol. 51, page 64 (1897), LACA; "At the Court House: The Council Wins," *Los Angeles Times*, April 23, 1897; "All Along the Line," *Los Angeles Times*, November 4, 1897; "City Government," *Los Angeles Times*, January 1, 1898; "The Pie Distributed," *Los Angeles Times*, January 4, 1899; *HDAR* (1904): 21.
15. Mary K. Sedgwick, "Instructive District Nursing," *Forum* 22 (1896): 302.
16. Lillian D. Wald, *The House on Henry Street* (New York: Henry Holt, 1915), 445. See also Lillian D. Wald, "The Henry Street (The Nurses) Settlement, New York," *Charities* 16 (April 7, 1906): 35; "Twenty Years of It in the Henry Street Nurses' Settlement," *Survey* 31 (February 14, 1914): 608. See also Karen Buhler-Wilkerson, *No Place Like Home*, 98–113.
17. "A Settlement in Adobe," *The Commons*, May 1897, 3.
18. Katharine Coman, "Casa Castelar," *The Commons* 13 (January 1903): 13; the Los Angeles Settlement Association, *The College Settlement*, 8 and 10.
19. See *IDNR* (1898–1907): 18; *IDNR* (1907–1908): 5; *IDNR* (1908–1910): 20; *IDNR* (1910–1911): 22; *IDNR* (1911–1912): 29; *IDNR* (1912–1913): 8.
20. The Los Angeles Settlement Association, *The College Settlement*, 10.
21. Maude B. Foster, "The Settlement and Socialism," *The Commons*, May 1899.
22. Ibid.
23. Sherry Katz estimates that there were hundreds of female members of the Socialist Party of California. See Katz, "Dual Commitments," 106 and 138, fn. 11.
24. Material for this section comes from City Archives Petition No. 683 (1899), LACA; City Archives Petition No. 189 (1901), LACA; Los Angeles City Directory, 1899 and 1901; see also "Not a Nuisance," *Los Angeles Times*, September 27, 1899; "Report of the Police Commission: Settlement Upheld," *Los Angeles Times*, September 27, 1899; "Trouble Ahead for Reformers," *Los Angeles Times*, February 10, 1901; "Many Measures Passed by the Council," *Los Angeles Times*, March 19, 1901; "College Settlement Was Under Fire," *Los Angeles Times*, March 24, 1901.
25. The council turned the issue over to the Finance Committee in 1899 and to the Police Commission in 1901.
26. City Council Minutes, vol. 60, page 274 (1901), LACA.
27. Evelynn Hammonds, *Childhood's Deadly Scourge*, especially chapter 4. Nancy Tomes, *The Gospel of Germs: Men, Women, and the Microbe in American Life* (Cambridge, Mass.: Harvard University Press, 1998).
28. I cannot date with greater specificity when the city health department changed its classification system because it did not publish annual reports between 1890 and 1904.

29. It should be noted that Hammonds's work on diphtheria demonstrates that physicians did not easily reconcile the privileging of the lab over experiential knowledge. See Hammonds, *Childhood's Deadly Scourge*.
30. Alice O'Connor, *Poverty Knowledge: Social Science, Social Policy, and the Poor in Twentieth-Century U.S. History* (Princeton, N. J.: Princeton University Press, 2001), chapter 1.
31. Bureau of the Census, *Population by Sex, General Nativity, and Color for Places Having 2,500 Inhabitants* (Washington, D.C.: Bureau of the Census, 1900). This figure is based on the enumeration of Wards 2, 7, 8, and 9, where the majority of the association's patients resided.
32. *IDNR* (1911–1912): 15.
33. Regarding shifting perceptions, see George Sanchez, "Go after the Women: Americanization and the Mexican Immigrant Woman, 1915–1929," in *Unequal Sisters: A Multicultural Reader in U.S. Women's History*, ed. Ellen DuBois and Vicki Ruíz (New York: Routledge, 1990); see also Abel, *Tuberculosis and the Politics of Exclusion*; Deverell, *Whitewashed Adobe*, chapter five; Molina, *Fit to Be Citizens?*
34. See Douglas Monroy, *Rebirth: Mexican Los Angeles from the Great Migration to the Great Depression* (Berkeley: University of California Press, 1990), 83–87; Sanchez, *Becoming Mexican American*, 20.
35. On the discourse of "city profitable" versus "city livable," see Maureen A. Flanagan, "The City Profitable, the City Livable: Environmental Policy, Gender, and Power in Chicago in the 1910s," *Journal of Urban History* 22, no. 2 (1996): 163–190.
36. Judging by Yssabella Waters's statistical tables, it does not appear that carfare was an unusual perk. Still, the NOPHN looked to Los Angeles for auto advice; see "Transportation," *The Public Health Nurse* 17, no. 1 (1925): 105.
37. Although I began this chapter using Maude Foster's maiden name, I have chosen to switch at this point in the chapter and refer to Foster by her married name in discussing her management of LACSA's public health nursing program because it is the name by which she signed all of her printed annual reports.
38. See "Events in Society," *Los Angeles Times*, July 1, 1902, "Marriage Licenses," *Los Angeles Times*, June 29, 1902. Although he appears to have grown up in a comfortable setting, Nathan Weston did not share his wife's elite background. See U.S. Census Manuscript 1870.
39. I am indebted to Marianne Peterson and Jane Weller, descendants of Anna Foster, who generously shared family information with me (phone conversation with Marianne Peterson, October 18, 1997 and letter to the author from Jane Weller, December 22, 1997.)
40. Ernest K. Foster's California Biography, Los Angeles Public Library. William A. Spalding, *History of Los Angeles* (Los Angeles: J. R. Finnell and Sons, 1931), vol. 3, 144–145. U.S. Census Manuscripts for Jno W. Foster, 1870, Pittsburgh, 4th Ward, page 80, line 20; Bella Foster, 1880, Pittsburgh, e.d. 104, line 9; Samuel F. Hammond, 1900, Pittsburgh, e.d. 240, line 14; Samuel F. Hammond, 1910, Los Angeles, e.d., 180, family 3.
41. "Society: Settlements Association," *Los Angeles Times*, December 8, 1895.
42. *First Report of the Los Angeles Settlements Association*, 9 and 32. The settlement established La Primavera Club to train young men in citizenship and teach them English.
43. *First Report of the Los Angeles Settlements Association*, 26–30.
44. Jean Glasscock, *Wellesley College, 1875–1975: A Century of Women* (Wellesley, Mass.: Wellesley College, 1975), 136. See also *Wellesley College Calendar*, 1883–1884.

45. The term "Lady Manager" was ubiquitous in this period. See, for instance, Ruth Crocker, *Mrs. Russell Sage: Women's Activism and Philanthropy in Gilded Age and Progressive Era America* (Bloomington: Indiana University Press, 2006), chapter 6.
46. Weston's college education might have muted the types of conflicts Buhler-Wilkerson found between lady managers and leaders of nursing. See Buhler-Wilkerson, *No Place Like Home*, 29–35; Buhler-Wilkerson, *False Dawn*, 48.
47. "In Social Spheres," *Los Angeles Times*, April 21, 1889.
48. I determined this by comparing the *First Report of the Los Angeles Settlements Association*, Names of Donations, Including Associate Memberships, from February 1894 to February 1897, with "In Social Spheres: The Wellesley Club," *Los Angeles Times*, July 16, 1896. See also "In Social Spheres: Collegiate Alumnae Reception," *Los Angeles Times*, May 16, 1894; "In Social Spheres: A Luncheon," *Los Angeles Times*, January 14, 1896; "Society," *Los Angeles Times*, January 27, 1897.
49. "New Work of the Settlement," *Los Angeles Times*, July 10, 1904.
50. Waters, *Visiting Nursing in the United States*, 19. Janis Appier found that Los Angeles's first policewomen donned simple white dresses because they resembled that of nurses. She suggests that this denoted their subordinate status within the city's law enforcement system. At the same time, this resemblance gave public health nurses a measure of authority. Appier, *Policing Women*, 63. My thanks to Anastasia J. Christman for drawing my attention to this reference.
51. For LACSA's mission statement, see Woods, *Handbook of Settlements*, 11.
52. *IDNR* (1898–1907): 23.
53. *IDNR* (1911–1912): 12.
54. *IDNR* (1898–1907): 3.
55. *IDNR* (1908–1910): 5.
56. See Lisbeth Haas, *Conquests and Historical Identities in California, 1769–1936* (Berkeley: University of California Press, 1995); Deverell, *Whitewashed Adobe*, chapter 6; Douglas Monroy, *Thrown among Strangers: The Making of Mexican Culture in Frontier California* (Berkeley: University of California Press, 1993); Leonard Pitt, *Decline of the Californios: A Social History of the Spanish-Speaking Californias, 1846–1890* (Berkeley: University of California Press, 1999).
57. *IDNR* (1911–1912): 15.
58. Ibid., 11 and 15.
59. "A House-Warming," *Los Angeles Times*, March 4, 1898.
60. *IDNR* (1911–1912): 11.
61. *IDNR* (1908–1910): 8–13 and 22.
62. *IDNR* (1911–1912): 11.
63. Letter from Alice M. Halloran to Jean F. McNair dated October 20, 1905, Box 39, McNair Family Papers, Huntington Library.
64. *IDNR* (1908–1910): 6 and 8–9.
65. *IDNR* (1911–1912): 7 and 9.
66. Reverby, *Ordered to Care*, 1–7.
67. *IDNR* (1911–1912): 8.
68. *IDNR* (1908–1910): 9–10.
69. Using a comparative consumer price index, $7,000 would have been worth $87,000 in 2007 (www.measuringworth.com).
70. The stories in this section come from *IDNR* (1908–1910): 9, 11–12.
71. The Los Angeles Humane Society for Children was "organized and conducted for the prevention of cruelty to children." See Box 28, Folder 5, Caroline Severance Collection, Huntington Library.

72. On the history of the College of Medicine, see George Kress, *A History of the Medical Profession of Southern California* (Los Angeles: Press of the Times-Mirror Print. and Binding House, 1910), 70–83; Viola Lockhart Warren, "The Old College of Medicine," *Historical Society of Southern California Quarterly*, December 1959–March 1960. Limited archival records of the College of Medicine are located at the UCLA University Archives and the Huntington Library.
73. Kress, *A History*, 71.
74. Abraham Flexner, *Medical Education in the United States and Canada* (New York: Carnegie Foundation, 1910), 189.
75. *IDNR* (1898–1907): 19.
76. *IDNR* (1908–1910): 8.
77. Woods, *Handbook of Settlements*, 10.
78. *IDNR* (1898–1907): 10.
79. Mary J. Workman, "Brownson House Settlement Work," *The Tidings* 16, no. 51 (1910): 77.
80. *IDNR* (1898–1907): 20; *IDNR* (1907–1908): 4; *IDNR* (1911–1912): 14.
81. *IDNR* (1908–1910), 10.
82. The Los Angeles Settlement Association, *The College Settlement*, 14.
83. *HDAR* (1904): 7.
84. The Los Angeles Settlement Association, *The College Settlement*, 12.
85. *IDNR* (1898–1907): 8.
86. *HDAR* (1904): 7.
87. "Board of Health: Wants More School Nurses," *Los Angeles Times*, July 6, 1904.
88. Waters, *Visiting Nursing in the United States*, 367.
89. The Los Angeles Settlement Association, *The College Settlement*, 12–13; *IDNR* (1907–1908): 4; *HDAR* (1911): 61.
90. City Archives Petition No. 650 (1897), LACA.
91. Board of Health Minutes, February 15, 1910, LACA.
92. "Measles Rage; Children Die," *Los Angeles Times*, November 3, 1909.
93. Ibid.
94. Leavitt, *The Healthiest City*, 98–107.
95. *IDNR* (1908–1910): 5.
96. "Measles Rage; Children Die," *Los Angeles Times*, November 3, 1909.
97. *IDNR* (1908–1910):16.
98. *IDNR* (1910–1911): 7.
99. Board of Health Minutes, December 30, 1909, LACA.
100. Board of Health Minutes, January 18, 1910, LACA.
101. Board of Health Minutes, January 31, 1910, LACA.
102. Board of Health Minutes, August 17, 1909; August 31, 1909; December 30, 1909; January 31, 1910; February 15, 1910, LACA.
103. Sirch had trained at the Buffalo General Hospital Training School and worked in Buffalo's District Nursing Program. See *HDAR* (1911): 61–62; Margaret F. Sirch's Registration with the State Board of Health as a Public Health Nurse. California State Board of Health, 1920 (Public Health—Nursing App. 1920–1928. California State Archives).
104. *HDAR* (1913): 84.
105. *IDNR* (1912–1913); "A House-Warming," *Los Angeles Times*, March 4, 1898.
106. FMC member Ada M. Davidson served for seven years, six as president. Other FMC members included Julia R. Johnson, who was a physician, and Mary A. Boynton.

107. *HDAR* (1915): 108.
108. *HDAR* (1919): 47–48.
109. Brainard, *Evolution of Public Health Nursing*, 257–259.
110. Buhler-Wilkerson, *False Dawn*, 111–115.

Chapter 2: Public Authority for a Private Program

1. *Report of the Housing Commission of the City of Los Angeles* (1906–1908), 3 (hereafter *HCR*).
2. Scholars also approach the historical topic as a multifaceted one that intersected with issues of class and gender. Christman, "The Best Laid Plans," 176–178; Paul Groth, *Living Downtown: The History of Residential Hotels in the United States* (Berkeley: University of California Press, 1994), especially chapters 7 and 8; Joanne J. Meyerowitz, *Women Adrift: Independent Wage Earners in Chicago, 1880–1930* (Chicago: University of Chicago Press, 1988), 79–90.
3. Jacob Riis, "The Tenement: The Real Problem of Civilization," *The Forum* 19 (1895): 83.
4. Gwendolyn Wright, *Building the Dream: A Social History of Housing in America* (Cambridge, Mass.: MIT Press, [1981] 1993): 124–125.
5. My work supports that of William Deverell and Natalia Molina, who analyze the various ways civic boosters and public health officials used the fact that Mexicans occupied the house courts to dismiss the possibility of improving these structures. However, I also look at female reformers and their inclusion of a variety of working-class immigrants in conceptualizing public health policies. Deverell, *Whitewashed Adobe*, chapter 5; Natalia Molina, "Illustrating Cultural Authority: Medicalized Representations of Mexican Communities in Early-Twentieth-Century Los Angeles," *Aztlán* 28(1) (2003): 129–143; see also Monroy, *Rebirth*, 23–25, and David Ward, *Poverty, Ethnicity, and the American City, 1840–1920: Changing Conceptions of the Slum and the Ghetto* (New York: Cambridge University Press, 1989).
6. Nancy Tomes, "The Private Side of Public Health: Sanitary Science, Domestic Hygiene, and the Germ Theory, 1870–1900," *Bulletin of the History of Medicine* 64 (4) (1990): 509–539.
7. Bureau of the Census, *Population of the Fifty Largest Cities at Each Census from 1840 to 1910. Arranged in the Order of Their Rank* (Washington, D.C: Bureau of the Census, 1910).
8. See, for instance, Fogelson, *The Fragmented Metropolis*, 161, and Carey McWilliams, *Southern California: An Island on the Land* (Layton, Utah: Peregrine Smith Book, 1946; reprint 1994), 360–361.
9. U.S. Bureau of the Census 1890, "Table 19—Population by Sex, General Nativity, and Color, of Places Having 25,000 Inhabitants or More: 1890," page 451; U.S. Bureau of the Census 1900, "Table 23—Population by Sex, General Nativity, and Color, of Places Having 25,000 Inhabitants or More: 1900," page 609.
10. John H. M. Laslett, "Historical Perspectives: Immigrants and the Rise of a Distinctive Urban Region, 1900–1970," in *Ethnic Los Angeles*, ed. Roger Waldinger and Mehdi Bozorgmehr (New York: Russell Sage Foundation, 1996), 41–47; Sánchez, *Becoming Mexican American*, 75–77.
11. *HCR* (1906–1908): 4–5.
12. "Selections from Records of the Friday Morning Club of Los Angeles" [essay], 1895, page 6, Box 1, Folder 11; Friday Morning Club (Los Angeles), Caroline Severance Collection, Huntington Library.

13. Gullett, *Becoming Citizens*, chapter 2.
14. *First Report of the Work of the Los Angeles Settlements Association at Casa de Castelar*, 2–3.
15. William T. Elsing, "Life in New York Tenement-Houses as Seen by a City Missionary," *Scribner's Magazine* 11, no. 73 (1892): 701.
16. Deverell, *Whitewashed Adobe*, 133–135. In an ironic twist, LACSA's first residence was in an adobe. "A Settlement in Adobe," *The Commons* 2, no. 1 (April–May 1897): 3–4.
17. *First Report of the Work of the Los Angeles Settlements Association at Casa de Castelar*, 2–6.
18. *HDAR* (1890): 3, 4, and 7–9.
19. Molina, "Contested Bodies and Cultures," 1–2.
20. *HDAR* (1890): 20.
21. The first published account of Riis's remark appeared in the Housing Commission of the City of Los Angeles's first report in 1908, three years after his visit. On the repetition of the comment, see Walter Wright Alley, *A Brief History of Public Housing Activities in Los Angeles* (Los Angeles: Los Angeles Municipal Housing Commission, 1936), 1; William H. Matthews, "The House Courts of Los Angeles," *The Survey*, July 5, 1913, 461; Ricardo Romo, "Mexican Workers in the City: Los Angeles, 1915–1930" (Ph.D. diss., UCLA, 1975), 82; George Sanchez, *Becoming Mexican American*, 75.
22. James B. Lane, *Jacob R. Riis and the American City* (New York: National University Publications Kennikat Press, 1974), 146.
23. Woods, *Handbook of Settlements*, 11–12.
24. "New Energy, More Work," *Los Angeles Times*, December 9, 1906.
25. "Life in the Slums of the Great Metropolis," *Los Angeles Examiner*, January 4, 1905; "Jacob A. Riis on Slum and Paradise," *Los Angeles Times*, January 4, 1905.
26. "Riis to Speak Again," *Los Angeles Herald*, January 4, 1905.
27. "Jacob Riis Tells of 'Tony,' Child of the Slums," *Los Angeles Herald*, January 8, 1905.
28. "Jacob A. Riis on Slum and Paradise," *Los Angeles Times*, January 4, 1905; "Heart of Riis Ever Is Open," *Los Angeles Times*, January 8, 1905.
29. Letter from Jacob Riis to Lyman Powell, December 1904; letter from Jacob Riis to Lyman Powell, March 1905, The Jacob A. Riis Collection, New York Public Library (hereafter NYPL).
30. Riis attempted to rest at Miradero Sanitarium, an institution restricted to nontubercular patients. See Lane, *Jacob R. Riis*, 176. See also letter from E. P. Leiford to Jacob Riis, March 28, 1905, Jacob A. Riis Collection, Library of Congress (hereafter LC).
31. "Jacob A. Riis on Slum and Paradise," *Los Angeles Times*, January 4, 1905.
32. The standard percentage on real estate investments in southern California was 6 to 7 percent. See the "Money Wanted" section in the classifieds in the *Los Angeles Times*, February 1, 1905, and the "Money" section in the classifieds of the *Los Angeles Herald*, January 31, 1905.
33. Alley, *A Brief History*, 1; Matthews, "House Courts," 461.
34. There was some overlap between the WCF and LACSA; Evelyn Stoddart, a founding member of LACSA, served on the board of directors for WCF. See "Women's Clubs," *Los Angeles Times*, October 4, 1905.
35. "Women's Clubs," *Los Angeles Times*, March 1, 1905; "Are Aroused over Garbage" *Los Angeles Times*, March 29, 1905; "Women Join Forces against Disgrace," *Los Angeles Times*, February 28, 1905; "War on Slums to Be Pressed," *Los Angeles Times*, September 7, 1906; "Women's Clubs," *Los Angeles Times*, October 1, 1905.

36. "Some of the Dangerous Sanitary Conditions Discovered in New Los Angeles Slums," *Los Angeles Times*, October 1, 1905.
37. August 12, 1905–August 15, 1905, Diary 1904–1905, Box 3: Diaries, 1886–1910, Graham Taylor Papers, Newberry Library, Chicago, Illinois.
38. "At the Churches Yesterday," *Los Angeles Times*, August 7, 1905, page 16; "Brevities," *Los Angeles Times*, August 12, 1905.
39. To understand how his illness impacted his perceptions of public health, see Emily K. Abel, *Suffering in the Land of Sunshine: A Los Angeles Illness Narrative* (New Brunswick, N.J.: Rutgers University Press, 2006). See also Donald Ray Culton, "Charles Dwight Willard: Los Angeles City Booster and Professional Reformer, 1888–1914" (Ph.D. diss., University of Southern California, 1971).
40. August 15, 1905, Diary 1904–1905, Box 3: Diaries, 1886–1910, Graham Taylor Papers, Newberry Library, Chicago, Illinois.
41. "At the Churches Yesterday," *Los Angeles Times*, August 14, 1905.
42. "'Don't Crowd Your Taste.' Dr. Graham Taylor Tendered Reception," *Los Angeles Times*, August 16, 1905.
43. Groth, *Living Downtown*, 208–216.
44. DeForest and Veiller, *The Tenement House Problem*, xxix.
45. "Some of the Dangerous Sanitary Conditions Discovered in New Los Angeles Slums," *Los Angeles Times*, October 1, 1905.
46. Bessie B. Stoddart, "The Courts of Sonoratown," *Charities and the Commons* 15, no. 9 (1905): 295–299.
47. *Municipal Affairs*, September 1905. See also Fogelson, *The Fragmented Metropolis*, 98, 233, 236, 249–250.
48. "Fight the 'Slums,'" *Los Angeles Times*, February 14, 1906.
49. Originally from Ohio, Mary Adair Veeder was single, educated, and thirty years old when she relocated to Los Angeles with her aunt, Abby C. Adair, in 1895. A few years later Veeder's six-year-old cousin, Margaret Mackay, came to live with them. They were not without means, as indicated by the fact that they were able to hire a domestic servant. The census always listed Veeder's occupation as "none," which leads me to believe that she did not pursue any career other than settlement work. Although it is unclear exactly when Veeder became involved with LACSA, by 1905 she was on the board of directors and an executive of its membership committee. See *Los Angeles City Directory*, 1895, and United States Census Manuscript 1900, 1910, 1920, and 1930; the Los Angeles Settlement Association, *The College Settlement*, 19. Titian James Coffey graduated from the local College of Medicine in 1898 and worked for many years with LACSA advising them on maternity issues. According to Lee M. A. Simpson, attorney Elizabeth Kenney was "the most prolific advocate for women's property rights" in California. See Lee M. A. Simpson, *Selling the City: Gender, Class, and the California Growth Machine, 1880–1940* (Stanford, Calif.: Stanford University Press, 2004), 47. George E. Bergstrom was responsible for a number of beaux arts buildings erected in the downtown area. He was also the founder of the nonprofit Allied Architects Association. See "The Allied Architects Association of Los Angeles," *Western Architect*, August 1921, 85–86. *National Cyclopedia of American Biography*, 368–369. (I am indebted to Gail Ostergren for drawing my attention to these sources.) Reverend William Horace Day received his theological training at the Yale Divinity School and the Chicago Theological Seminary. In 1900, he moved to Los Angeles to become a co-pastor with his father. See "Rev. William Horace Day," *Los Angeles Express*, May 4, 1912.

50. Lubove, *The Progressives and the Slums*, 26.
51. *HCR* (1910–1913): 11.
52. *HCR* (1908–1909): 12.
53. *HCR* (1906–1908): 7 and 10.
54. Ibid., 10.
55. *HCR* (1909–1910): 12.
56. *HCR* (1906–1908): 12.
57. *HCR* (1910–1913): 20–21.
58. DeForest, *The Tenement House Problem*, 385–417.
59. Elsing, "Life in New York Tenement-Houses," 718.
60. "War on Slums to Be Pressed," *Los Angeles Times*, September 7, 1906.
61. Fred W. Viehe, "The First Recall: Los Angeles Urban Reform or Machine Politics?" *Southern California Quarterly* 70, no. 1 (1988): 1–28.
62. "War on Slums to Be Pressed," *Los Angeles Times*, September 7, 1906.
63. Los Angeles's total population in 1900 was 102,479. The Sixth Ward had 14,044 people living in it. It had 11,587 native whites, 2,457 foreign-born whites, 335 African Americans, and 80 Chinese. See Bureau of the Census, *Population by Sex, General Nativity, and Color* (Washington, D.C.: Bureau of the Census, 1900).
64. "War on the Slums Now to Be Pressed," *Los Angeles Times*, September 7, 1906; "Housing Problem Too Much for Volunteers," *Los Angeles Express*, October 16, 1906.
65. "Women's Clubs," *Los Angeles Times*, November 17, 1906.
66. Board of Health Minutes, November 22, 1906, LACA; "Housing Ordinance," *Los Angeles Times*, November 23, 1906.
67. "Council Passes Slum Ordinance," *Los Angeles Express*, February 4, 1907.
68. Matthews, "The House Courts," 464.
69. George W. Gillette, "The Tenement Situation in Buffalo," *Charities and the Commons* 17 (1906): 70–73.
70. *Municipal Affairs*, May 1907, 1–2.
71. *HCR* (1906–1908): 16.
72. *HCR* (1906–1908): 12.
73. For another example, see George J. Sanchez, "Go After the Women," 284–297.
74. Letters to the *Times, Los Angeles Times*, October 28, 1913.
75. *HCR* (1906–1908): 25.
76. See, for instance, a discussion of Chicago in "Women as Tenement House Inspectors," *Charities and the Commons* 15, no. 24 (1906): 864–865. See also Emily Wayland Dinwiddle, "Sanitary Inspection by the Visiting Nurse," *Visiting Nurse Quarterly* 4, no. 2 (January 1912): 29–34; Lawrence Veiller, "A Programme of Housing Reform," in *Housing Problems in America: Proceedings of the First National Conference on Housing*.
77. Letter from Riis to Dr. [Jane E.] Robbins dated January 15, 1907 (LC).
78. "Riis to Lecture Here," *Los Angeles Times*, February 2, 1907; "Slum Warrior Sounds Alarm," *Los Angeles Times*, February 7, 1907; "Riis Tells of Work in Slums," *Los Angeles Herald*, February 7, 1907.
79. Jacob A. Riis, "America's Civic Awakening," *Charities and the Commons* 19 (1908): 1600; see also Jacob A. Riis, "Heading Off the Slums in the West," *Charities and the Commons* 19 (1908), 1703–1706.
80. "To Eradicate Slums" *Los Angeles Times*, August 8, 1907.
81. Board of Health Minutes, December 1, 1903; July 17, 1907; August 7, 1907, LACA.

82. "Queirolo's Turn," *Los Angeles Times*, December 15, 1908.
83. "Rubbing Out Plague Spots," *Los Angeles Times*, August 29, 1907.
84. "Women's Clubs," *Los Angeles Times*, March 10, 1908.
85. *HCR* (1906–1908): 19.
86. Ibid., 6, 23.
87. "Women's Clubs," *Los Angeles Times*, March 3, 1908.
88. "Slum Courts Disappearing," *Los Angeles Times*, August 30, 1908; "Capital for House Court," *Los Angeles Times*, September 6, 1908.
89. *HCR* (1908–1909): 6.
90. Ibid., 4.
91. *HCR* (1908–1909): 6.
92. Ibid.
93. *HCR* (1908–1909): 12.
94. *HCR* (1906–1908): 24–25.
95. Mrs. Vladimir Piatnizky, Baroness Johanna Von Wagner, was born in Krefeld, Germany. She moved to the United States when she became a widow. She began her training at McLean Hospital in Boston and completed a course in sanitation at Columbia University. See "Piatnizky Obsequies at Lomita," *Los Angeles Times*, September 16, 1926; "Woman Comes to Aid Poor," *Los Angeles Times*, December 13, 1908; *HCR* (1908–1909): 20 and 22.
96. "A Woman Worker in the Tenements," *Los Angeles Times*, May 18, 1902.
97. *HCR* (1908–1909): 12, 14, and 22.
98. "Woman Comes to Aid Poor," *Los Angeles Times*, December 13, 1908.
99. *HCR* (1910–1913): 20.
100. *HCR* (1908–1909): 14.
101. *HCR* (1910–1913): 19.
102. "Poor People Preyed Upon," *Los Angeles Times*, July 19, 1909.
103. "Charity Workers Meet," *Los Angeles Times*, January 19, 1910.
104. "Model Village Stands Alone," *Los Angeles Times*, December 9, 1910.
105. See Box 54, folder "Municipal Housing Association," John Randolph Haynes Papers (Collection 1241), Department of Special Collections, University Research Library, University of California, Los Angeles.
106. *HCR* (1910–1913): 13.
107. Ibid., 10.
108. *HCR* (1909–1910): 11–12; *HCR* (1908–1909): 16.
109. *HCR* (1908–1909): 10.
110. *HDAR* (1914): 128–129.
111. *HCR* (1910–1913): 23–24.
112. City Archives Petitions No. 1411 (1912), LACA. Other than referring the petition to the Public Welfare Committee, the city council minutes do not indicate any action upon the petition. City Council Minutes, vol. 89, page 247. Regarding the Armstrongs, see the 1900 U.S. Census and 1911 city directory.
113. City Council Minutes, vol. 91, page 581, LACA.
114. *HDAR* (1910): 69–70.
115. "New Status for Housing Board," *Los Angeles Times*, April 13, 1913; "Lack of Funds Is Complaint," *Los Angeles Times*, May 10, 1913.
116. *HCR* (1910–1913), 65.
117. Letter from John Ihdler to Phillips, July 25, 1912, Box 2, Folder 2, Katherine Philips Edson Papers, Charles E. Young Research Library, Department of Special

Collections, University of California, Los Angeles. My thanks to Anastasia Christman for bringing this source to my attention.
118. On the haziness of defining apartments and tenements, see Wright, *Building the Dream*, 135.
119. *HDAR* (1914): 126.
120. *HDAR* (1914): 123.
121. *HDAR* (1916): 106.
122. Molina, "Illustrating Cultural Authority," 129–143.
123. See Emory S. Bogardus, "The House-Court Problem," *American Journal of Sociology* 22, no. 3 (1916): 391–399; Elizabeth Fuller, "The Mexican Housing Problem in Los Angeles," in *The Near Side of the Mexican Question*, ed. J. S. Stowell (New York: George H. Doran, 1921); Gladys Patric, *Study of the Housing and Social Conditions in the Ann Street District of Los Angeles California* (Los Angeles: Los Angeles Society for the Study and Prevention of Tuberculosis, 1916).

Chapter 3: Bovines, Babies, and Bacteriology

1. See Edwards, *Angels in the Machinery*; Gullett, *Becoming Citizens*, 181–191; Katz, "Socialist Women and Progressive Reform."
2. Duffy, *The Sanitarians*, 183–185; Leavitt, *The Healthiest City*, chapter 5; Richard Meckel, *Save the Babies: American Public Health Reform and the Prevention of Infant Mortality, 1850–1929* (Baltimore: Johns Hopkins University Press, 1990), 63–65; Charles E. North, "Milk and Its Relation to Public Health," in *A Half Century of Public Health*, ed. Mazÿck P. Ravenel (New York: American Public Health Association, 1921).
3. Fred Bateman, "Improvement in American Dairy Farming, 1850–1910: A Quantitative Analysis," *Journal of Economic History* 28 (June 1968): 255–273; Daniel Ralston Block, "The Development of Regional Institutions in Agriculture: The Chicago Milk Marketing Order" (Ph.D. diss., UCLA, 1997); Gordon J. Fielding, "The Los Angeles Milkshed: A Study of the Political Factor in Agriculture," *Geographical Review* 54 (January 1964): 1–12; Sally McMurry, *Transforming Rural Life: Dairying Families and Agricultural Change, 1820–1885* (Baltimore: Johns Hopkins University Press, 1995); Thomas R. Pegram, "Public Health and Progressive Dairying in Illinois," *Agricultural History* 65 (Winter 1991): 36–50; Thomas Ross Pirtle, *History of the Dairy Industry* (Chicago: Mojonnier Bros., 1926); Robert L. Santos, "Dairying in California through 1910," *Southern California Quarterly* 76 (Summer 1994): 175–194.
4. Block, "The Development of Regional Institutions," 46–49.
5. City Archives Petition No. 1906 (1920), LACA.
6. U.S. Bureau of the Census, 1900, "Table 42: Number of Specified Domestic Animals to 100,000 Inhabitants in Certain Cities and Groups of Cities, June 1, 1900, Arranged According to Population."
7. Ordinance No. 16,985, LACA. The city amended the ordinance twice over the next four years; see Ordinance No. 19,040, and Ordinance No. 33,669. Although these regulations severely limited the number of urban cows, those individuals living in the oldest part of the city were still allowed to keep one cow.
8. City Archives Petition No. 2571 (1915), LACA.
9. This would have been worth approximately $6,000 in 2006 (www.measuringworth.com).
10. *HDAR* (1912): 50–55.

11. City Council Minutes, vol. 60, page 62; City Council Minutes, vol. 60, page 65, LACA. Communication from J. L. Stout filed February 11, 1901; affidavit of Guy Peterson, February 14, 1901; affidavit of Thomas Vestal, February 13, 1901, LACA.
12. "To Secure Better Food," *Los Angeles Times*, January 10, 1899.
13. Board of Health Minutes, October 10, 1906, LACA; "Defies Inspectors," *Los Angeles Times*, August 8, 1907.
14. Board of Health Minutes, September 21, 1905, LACA.
15. "One More Pure Milk Crusade," *Los Angeles Times*, August 29, 1905.
16. Naomi Rogers, *Dirt and Disease: Polio before FDR* (New Brunswick, N.J.: Rutgers University Press, 1992); Tomes, *Gospel of Germs*.
17. "Top-Notchers in the Milk," *Los Angeles Times*, September 4, 1909.
18. "Milky Way Dimmed," *Los Angeles Times*, November 16, 1900.
19. "Family Skeletons Put in the Milk," *Los Angeles Times*, February 28, 1902; "No Milk Trust," *Los Angeles Times*, February 15, 1903; "White Trust to Sell Milk," *Los Angeles Times*, December 9, 1904.
20. For instances, see ads in *Los Angeles Times*, February 1, 1908, and June 15, 1910.
21. *Los Angeles Times*, October 14, 1906
22. "Milk War Is Breaking Out," *Los Angeles Times*, April 15, 1902.
23. Regarding Mrs. Wilson's battle with Alpine Dairy, see "Widow Fights Milk 'Trust,'" *Los Angeles Times*, January 23, 1907, and "Milk, Not Blood, Runs in Rivers through Fierce War of Dealers and Ranchman," *Los Angeles Times*, February 3, 1907. Sally McCurry explains the process by which the dairy industry was defeminized. The case of Los Angeles, however, demonstrates the continued participation of women in small-scale dairy production and distribution. Besides Mrs. Wilson, the city directory lists eighteen women who advertised their wares between 1897 and 1915.
24. "He's after Milk Trust," *Los Angeles Times*, February 7, 1907; *Los Angeles Herald*, February 9, 1907.
25. "Government May Help," *Los Angeles Times*, February 8, 1907; *Los Angeles Herald*, February 8, 1907.
26. *Los Angeles Herald*, February 8, 1907.
27. "Pen Points," *Los Angeles Times*, February 17, 1907.
28. "We Are No Trust," *Los Angeles Times*, September 23, 1907.
29. "Milk, Not Blood, Runs in Rivers through Fierce War of Dealers and Ranchman," *Los Angeles Times*, February 3, 1907.
30. Board of Health Minutes, June 19, 1907, LACA.
31. Board of Health Minutes, August 17, 1909, LACA.
32. Board of Health Minutes, September 22, 1909, LACA; "For Purer Milk," *Los Angeles Times*, September 23, 1909.
33. Board of Health Minutes, January 30, 1911, LACA.
34. See Meckel, *Save the Babies*, chapter 3.
35. Rima D. Apple, *Mothers and Medicine: A Social History of Infant Feeding, 1890–1950* (Madison: University of Wisconsin Press, 1987); Janet Golden, *A Social History of Wet Nursing in America: From Breast to Bottle* (New York: Cambridge University Press, 1996); Wolf, *Don't Kill Your Baby*, 30–41.
36. Curry, *Modern Mothers in the Heartland*, 5.
37. On works that tend to portray women as uninterested in using science, see Schultz, *Constructing Urban Culture*, 16; Stradling, *Smokestacks and Progressives*, 3, 62, and 119–120. On new research that looks at women's interest in technology-based solutions, see Flanagan, *Seeing with Their Hearts*, 93–94 and 99–100; Howard L. Platt,

"Jane Addams and the Ward Boss Revisited: Class, Politics, and Public Health in Chicago, 1890–1930," *Environmental History* 5 (April 2000): 194–222.
38. Leavitt, *The Healthiest City*, 181. See also Julie Miller, "To Stop the Slaughter of the Babies: Nathan Straus and the Drive for Pasteurized Milk, 1893–1920," *New York History* 74 (April 1993): 158–184.
39. Meckel, *Save the Babies*, 81.
40. Manfred J. Waserman, "Henry L. Coit and the Certified Milk Movement in the Development of Modern Pediatrics," *Bulletin of the History of Medicine* 46 (July–August 1972): 359–390. In Los Angeles, only one certified dairy existed in 1912: the Arden Certified Dairy. Its delivery routes were limited and it cost 15 cents a quart. See *Monthly Report of the Health Department of the City of Los Angeles* (October 1911): 1–3 (hereafter *HDMR*); "Report of the Los Angeles County Medical Milk Association," *Southern California Practitioner* 26 (January 1911): 44–45.
41. Leavitt, *Healthiest City*, chapter 5; Meckel, *Save the Babies*, chapter 3; Wolf, *Don't Kill Your Baby*, chapter 2.
42. U.S. Treasury Department, "Public Health Reports Issued Weekly by the United States Public Health Service," *The Legal Phases of Milk Control* (Washington, D.C.: Government Printing Office, 1929), 3110–3116.
43. Jacqueline Braitman also discusses Edson's initial engagement with milk reform. However, she fails to discuss Edson's participation in the tuberculin test controversy of 1912. See Jacqueline R. Braitman, "Katherine Philips Edson: A Progressive-Feminist in California's Era of Reform" (Ph.D. diss., UCLA, 1988), chapter 2. Regarding biographical details of Edson's life, see Jacqueline R. Braitman, "A California Stateswoman: The Public Career of Katherine Philips Edson," *California History* 65 (June 1986): 82–95; "Katherine Philips Edson," *Pacific Empire Press Reporter*, May 1913. See Box 4, Folder 253-44, Katherine Philips Edson Papers, Charles E. Young Research Library, Department of Special Collections, University of California, Los Angeles (hereafter KPE Collection).
44. Sklar, *Florence Kelley*; Florence Kelley and Kathryn Kish Sklar, *Notes of Sixty Years: the Autobiography of Florence Kelley*. First Person Series, No. 1 (Chicago: Published for the Illinois Labor History Society by the C. H. Kerr Pub. Co., 1986).
45. Letter from Florence Kelley to Katherine Philips Edson, dated August 3, 1909, Box 2, Folder 253-21, KPE Collection.
46. Katherine Philips Edson, "A Pure Milk Campaign," *Federation Courier*, September 1910, 21.
47. Letter from Edson to Mrs. Thomas, dated December 30, 1913, Box 1, Folder 253-11, KPE Collection.
48. Nancy Cott, *The Bonds of Womanhood: "Women's Sphere" in New England, 1780–1935* (New Haven, Conn.: Yale University Press, 1977). On the extension of this ideology to justify women's participation in public policy, see Flanagan, "The City Profitable," 163–190; Suellen M. Hoy, "Municipal Housekeeping: The Role of Women in Improving Urban Sanitation Practices, 1880–1917," in *Pollution and Reform in American Cities, 1870–1930*, ed. Martin V. Melosi (Austin: University of Texas Press, 1980).
49. Letter from Edson to Mrs. Thomas, dated January 23, 1914, Box 1, Folder 253-12, KPE Collection.
50. Milton J. Rosenau, *The Milk Question* (Boston and New York: Houghton Mifflin, 1912), 12.
51. See Catherine Phelps Edson, "The Present Status," *Federation Courier*, April 1911, 8–9.

52. See *Readers' Guide to Periodical Literature*, 1905–1909, 1456–1457.
53. Judy Barrett Litoff, *American Midwives: 1860 to the Present* (Westport, Conn.: Greenwood, 1978), 93.
54. "Birth, Death, and Infant Mortality Data in Los Angeles since 1890," *The Bulletin* (1933), Box 83, Folder 14, Collection 1241, John Randolph Haynes Collection, Special Collections, University of California, Los Angeles.
55. "Deaths from Impure Milk," *Los Angeles Times*, October 1, 1909.
56. Edson, "A Pure Milk Campaign," 21.
57. Ibid. See also Braitman, "Katherine Philips Edson," 79.
58. Stella Walker Durham, "The Portland Pure Milk War: The Story of a Victory Won by a City's Housewives," *Good Housekeeping* 50 (April 1910): 518–520; Mabel Craft Deering, "What Any Woman's Club Can Do in Reforming the Milk Supply," *Good Housekeeping* 50 (May 1910): 645–646; William Ruthven Flint, "Clean Milk at Moderate Cost," *Good Housekeeping* 50 (June 1910): 765–769.
59. Edson, "A Pure Milk Campaign," 21.
60. "Mrs. Edson Urges Pure Milk Supply," *Los Angeles Express*, June 17, 1910; "Mrs. Edson Flays the City Charter," *Los Angeles Herald*, June 18, 1910.
61. Ibid.
62. "Mrs. Edson Flays the City Charter," *Los Angeles Herald*, June 18, 1910.
63. Frank N. Bauskett, "The Danger of the Use of Milk from Tuberculosis Cows," *American Homes and Gardens* 7 (September 1910): 356–357; United States Department of Agriculture, Bureau of Animal Industry, *The Unsuspected but Dangerously Tuberculous Cow*, by E. C. Schroeder (Washington, D.C.: Government Printing Office, 1907).
64. City Council Minutes, vol. 50, page 745 (1897), LACA.
65. J. M. Grange and C. H. Collins, "Bovine Tubercle Bacilli and Disease in Animals and Man," *Epidemiology and Infection* 92 (October 1987): 221–234; D. G. Pritchard, "A Century of Bovine Tuberculosis 1888–1988: Conquest and Controversy," *Journal of Comparative Pathology* 99 (November 1988): 357–399; United States Department of Agriculture, Bureau of Animal Industry, *Bovine Tuberculosis and Public Health*, by D. E. Salmon (Washington, D.C.: Government Printing Office, 1904); United States Department of Agriculture, Bureau of Animal Industry, *Milk and Its Products as Carriers of Tuberculosis Infection*, by E. C. Schroeder (Washington, D.C.: Government Printing Office, 1909); United States Department of Agriculture, Bureau of Animal Industry, *The Dissemination of Disease by Dairy Products and Methods for Prevention* (Washington, D.C.: Government Printing Office, 1910).
66. Board of Health Minutes, October 22, 1903, LACA.
67. See mortality report in *HDAR* (1911). *Los Angeles Municipal News*, May 8, 1912.
68. *HDMR* (October 1911): 2.
69. Tuberculin injected into an infected animal raised its temperature a few degrees for a few hours. Once identified, the cow was to be destroyed and autopsied because the infection could only be proven by a postmortem exam.
70. Georgina D. Feldberg, *Disease and Class: Tuberculosis and the Shaping of Modern North American Society* (New Brunswick, N.J.: Rutgers University Press, 1995), 55–80; Francis Marion Pottenger, *The Fight against Tuberculosis: An Autobiography* (New York: H. Shuman, 1952); Francis Marion Pottenger, *Tuberculin in Diagnosis and Treatment* (St. Louis, Mo.: C. V. Mosby, 1913).
71. "Councilmen Stand Ready to Aid Club Women in Their Campaign for Pure Milk in Los Angeles," *Los Angeles Record*, June 18, 1910.
72. Ibid.

73. *IDNR* (1911–1913): 13–14.
74. Board of Health Minutes, June 28, 1910, LACA.
75. "New Standards in Milk Test," *Los Angeles Times*, June 29, 1910. By early July, however, the board began to backtrack on strengthening standards. Board of Health Minutes, July 8, 1910, LACA.
76. Board of Health Minutes, July 5, 1910, LACA.
77. George H. Hart, "Dairying in California Compared to the East," *Proceedings of the Ninth Annual Conference of the American Association of Medical Milk Commissions Held at San Francisco, California, June 17, 18, and 19, 1915* (Cincinnati, 1916), 56–58.
78. Wolf, *Don't Kill Your Baby*, 66.
79. *HDAR* (1912): 55.
80. Board of Health Minutes, July 9, 1910, LACA.
81. *HDMR* (October 1911): 1.
82. This was slightly stricter than that advocated by government expert Milton J. Rosenau. Rosenau, *The Milk Question*, 195.
83. Los Angeles City Council Minutes, November 28, 1911, LACA. Unfortunately, the minutes do not detail the substance of their protest but it does list those who spoke: attorney W. H. Dehn, Mrs. S. R. T. Watson, P. H. Nienkanp, Mrs. W. P. Harrel, G. A. Cherry, R. B. Urmston, and Geo B. Miller, president of the Mutual Dairy Association.
84. *Los Angeles Times*, May 24, 1912; *Los Angeles Municipal News*, May 15, 1912.
85. John Schlebecker, *A History of Dairy Journalism in the United States, 1850–1910* (Madison: University of Wisconsin Press, 1957), 163 and 219. "A Few Late Ideas," *California Cultivator*, August 27, 1908, 201; "Milk Supply" *California Cultivator* October 8, 1908, 346; "The Economic Importance of Animal Tuberculosis," *California Cultivator*, October 22 1908, 394–395; "Tuberculin Test Reliable," *California Cultivator*, November 26, 1908, 516; "Tuberculosis," *California Cultivator*, April 7, 1910, 439; "Test with Tuberculin," *California Cultivator*, June 23, 1910, 739; "Tuberculin," *California Cultivator*, August 4, 1910, 104; "Tuberculosis," *California Cultivator*, December 29, 1910, 677; "Whose Loss?" *California Cultivator*, January 5, 1911, 11; "Primer on Bovine Tuberculosis," *California Cultivator*, April 27, 1911, 524; "Germs Detected in Milk," *California Cultivator*, June 29, 1911, 769; "Tuberculosis," *California Cultivator*, September 21, 1911, 278; "Throat Trouble-Tuberculin Test," *California Cultivator*, September 28, 1911, 305; "Bovine Tuberculosis," *California Cultivator*, January 11, 1912, 44.
86. Perhaps Sobieski viewed herself as continuing a long family legacy of social activism; members on her paternal side had advocated for abolition and temperance. See John Sobieski, *The Life-Story and Personal Reminiscences of Col. John Sobieski* (Shelbyville, Ill. : J. L. Douthit and Son, 1900), 172–178 and 229.
87. "Pure Milk Is Given New Impetus," *Los Angeles Examiner*, May 24, 1912.
88. Braitman, "A California Stateswoman," 86; Edwards, *Angels in the Machinery*, chapter 3; Gullett, *Becoming Citizens*, 188–190.
89. Regarding Locke, see *Who's Who in Los Angeles* (Los Angeles, 1926–1927) and obituary from *Los Angeles Herald*, February 14, 1933.
90. Gullett, *Becoming Citizens*, 192–200.
91. See Sara G. Garrett, "The Woman's City Club of Los Angeles," *Out West Magazine*, March 1916, 132–133.
92. For an analysis of the popularization of knowledge about disease through mass media, see Ziporyn Terra Diane, *Disease in the Popular American Press: The Case of Diphtheria, Typhoid Fever, and Syphilis, 1870–1920* (Westport, Conn.: Greenwood, 1988).

93. "The Tuberculin Test," *Los Angeles Municipal News*, May 8, 1912.
94. "The Tuberculin Test," *Los Angeles Municipal News*, May 22, 1912.
95. *Bulletin of the Los Angeles County Medical Society* 42 (January 5, 1912): 3.
96. For Edson's plea, see "Communication Regarding Tuberculosis Test," *Southern California Practitioner* 27 (May 1912): 236–237; for Hart, Powers, and Pottenger's appeals, see *Bulletin of the Los Angeles County Medical Society* 42 (March 1, 1912); 42 (April 19, 1912); 42 (May 3, 1912); 42 (May 17, 1912).
97. "The Tuberculin Test," *Los Angeles Municipal News*, April 24, 1912; "The Tuberculin Test," *Los Angeles Municipal News*, May 1, 1912; "The Tuberculin Test," *Los Angeles Municipal News*, May 15, 1912.
98. "City's Health vs. Dairy's Dollars War Cry of Campaign," *Los Angeles Examiner*, May 19, 1912.
99. "The Tuberculin Test," *Los Angeles Municipal News*, April 24, 1912.
100. *Los Angeles Examiner*, May 27, 1912. See listing for G. Bloomfield, 435 S. Mathews St. in the Los Angeles City Directory (1913).
101. "The Tuberculin Test," *Los Angeles Municipal News*, May 1, 1912.
102. "The Tuberculin Test," *Los Angeles Municipal News*, May 8, 1912.
103. Wolf, *Don't Kill Your Baby*, 59–64.
104. On the question of precedent, see "The Tuberculin Test," *Los Angeles Municipal News*, April 24, 1912; May 1, 1912; May 8, 1912; for Pottenger's response, see "The Tuberculin Test," *Los Angeles Municipal News*, May 15, 1912.
105. "Tuberculin Test for Cows Fair to All and Insures Safe Milk," *Los Angeles Herald*, May 25, 1912.
106. "The Tuberculin Test," *Los Angeles Municipal News*, April 24, 1912.
107. "The Tuberculin Test," *Los Angeles Municipal News*, May 15, 1912.
108. "The Tuberculin Test," *Los Angeles Citizen*, May 17, 1912.
109. "The Tuberculin Test," *Los Angeles Municipal News*, May 22, 1912.
110. "City's Health vs. Dairy's Dollars War Cry of Campaign," *Los Angeles Examiner*, May 19, 1912.
111. "The Tuberculin Test," *Los Angeles Municipal News*, May 8, 1912; "The Tuberculin Test," *Los Angeles Municipal News*, May 22, 1912.
112. "The Tuberculin Test," *Los Angeles Citizen*, May 17, 1912.
113. "City's Health vs. Dairy's Dollars War Cry of Campaign," *Los Angeles Examiner*, May 19, 1912.
114. "Pet and Slip at Big Plans," *Los Angeles Times*, May 24, 1912.
115. The *Los Angeles Herald* and the *Los Angeles Examiner* formally supported the law. The *Los Angeles Times* and *Los Angeles Express* expressed no formal opinion.
116. "Pastors Favor Law to Require Tuberculin Test," *Los Angeles Herald*, May 21, 1912; "Put the Baby above The Cow," *Los Angeles Herald*, May 22, 1912; "Citizens Give Approval to Tuberculin Test," *Los Angeles Herald*, May 24, 1912.
117. "Pure Milk Is Given New Impetus," *Los Angeles Examiner*, May 24, 1912.
118. "Tuberculin Test Fight Near End," *Los Angeles Herald*, May 23, 1912.
119. Records of Election Returns, December 5, 1904–December 8, 1920, LACA. Unfortunately there is no archival evidence to aid in determining the vote by gender, class, and ethnicity.
120. "Tuberculin Test and Hall Levy Voted Down," *Los Angeles Times*, May 29, 1912.
121. "Milk from Sick Cows," *Southern California Practitioner* 27 (June 1912): 277.
122. "The Tuberculin Test," *Los Angeles Municipal News*, May 29, 1912.

123. "City Hall and Tuberculin Test Loses by Light Vote," *Los Angeles Examiner*, May 29, 1912.
124. George H. Hart, "Tuberculosis," in *Proceedings of the Ninth Annual Conference of the American Association of Medical Milk Commissions Held at San Francisco, California June 17, 18, and 19, 1915* (Cincinnati, 1916), 58.
125. See questionnaire of December 1913 from an "Englishwoman" to Edson on the impact of enfranchisement of women, Box 1, Folder 253-24, KPE Collection. See also letter from Edson to Hiram Johnson dated April 7, 1914, Box 1, Folder 253-12, KPE Collection.
126. For a longer discussion of these politics, see Braitman, "Katherine Philips Edson," 100–105.
127. Hart, "Tuberculosis," 58.
128. *HDMR* (April 1917): 1.
129. Letter from Edson to Hiram Johnson dated April 7, 1914, Box 1, Folder 253-12, KPE Collection. On account of his wife's illness, Nathan Straus moved to Los Angeles in 1913. After a year's recuperation, the Strauses made a number of public appearances discussing Zionism and health. See "Women's Work, Women's Clubs," *Los Angeles Times* March 12, 1914 ; "Straus Reception," *Los Angeles Times*, March 21, 1914; Letters to the *Times, Los Angeles Times*, March 24, 1914; "Noted Philanthropists Given Notable Tribute," *Los Angeles Times*, March 23, 1914.

Chapter 4: Delivering the City's Children

1. Natalia Molina also analyzes these photographs but to discuss official representations of Mexicans as public health dangers. See Molina, "Illustrating Cultural Authority," 141–142.
2. A crucial question of historical inquiry has been what caused this precipitous decline of midwifery in the early twentieth century. See Charlotte G. Borst, *Catching Babies: The Professionalization of Childbirth, 1870–1920* (Cambridge, Mass.: Harvard University Press, 1995); Judith Walzer Leavitt, *Brought to Bed: Child Bearing in America, 1750–1950* (New York: Oxford University Press, 1986); Litoff, *American Midwives*. Most recently, Susan L. Smith and Diane C. Vecchio have looked at how immigrant communities melded modern science with the practice of midwifery. See Susan L. Smith, *Japanese American Midwives: Culture, Community, and Health Politics, 1880–1950* (Champaign: University of Illinois Press, 2005); Diane C. Vecchio, *Merchants, Midwives, and Laboring Women: Italian Migrants in Urban America* (Champaign: University of Illinois Press, 2006).
3. Litoff, *American Midwives*, 93.
4. Litoff, *American Midwives*, 108–112.
5. "Birth, Death, and Infant Mortality Data in Los Angeles since 1890," *The Bulletin*, 1933, Box 83, Folder 14, Collection 1241, John Randolph Haynes Collection, Special Collections, University of California, Los Angeles.
6. In Los Angeles, as elsewhere, infant morality rates differed by ethnicity and race. Until 1929, however, the city health department did not publish statistical information on these differences.
7. S. Josephine Baker, "Schools for Midwives," *American Journal of Obstetrics and Diseases of Women and Children*, 65 (1912): 256–270.
8. Fogelson, *The Fragmented Metropolis*, 79.
9. *HDAR* (1910): 6.
10. Litoff, *American Midwives*, 92–93.

11. "A New Obstetrical Forceps," *Southern California Practitioner* 7, no. 5 (1892): 206–207.
12. "An Obstetrical Section of the County Medical Association," *Southern California Practitioner* 21, no. 3 (1906): 135–136; "The Perineum," *Southern California Practitioner* 7, no. 6 (1892): 237–245.
13. "The So-Called Midwife," *Southern California Practitioner* 11, no. 1 (1896): 23.
14. "Wash Your Hands," *Southern California Practitioner* 2, no. 10 (1887): 386–387.
15. "The So-Called Midwife," 23.
16. "The Doctor in Obstetrics," *Southern California Practitioner*, 6, no. 12 (1891): 585–587.
17. "Gynecology in Southern California," *Southern California Practitioner* 2, no. 10 (1887): 310.
18. "Report of Obstetrical Cases," *Southern California Practitioner* 6, no. 11 (1891): 505–509.
19. Board of Health Minutes, February 20, 1889, LACA.
20. "Midwife Law Attacked," *Los Angeles Times*, April 9, 1904; Board of Health Minutes, July 27, 1901, LACA.
21. "Will Prosecute Fake Midwives," *Los Angeles Herald*, February 7, 1907. According to the 1920 United States Census Manuscript, Franco was sixty five years old. She and her husband, Carlos, owned their own home free of mortgage at 2446 East 1st Street. Three children lived with them. Her husband was a shoemaker, her son an automaker, and her daughter a fruit packer.
22. I have not found any archival record that would continue to provide individual information on midwife applications after the city disbanded its board of health in 1911.
23. *IDNR* (1898–1907): 21–24.
24. *IDNR* (1911–1912): 27.
25. "The Passing of the Midwife," *Southern California Practitioner* 15, no. 4 (1900): 113–114.
26. Charlotte G. Borst, "Teaching Obstetrics at Home: Medical Schools and Home Delivery Services in the First Half of the Twentieth Century," *Bulletin of the History of Medicine* 72 (1998): 220–245.
27. *IDNR* (1910–1911): 27.
28. *IDNR* (1907–1908): 3. Unfortunately, the name of the first maternity nurse is illegible.
29. *IDNR* (1910–1911): 18–19. Regarding comparative wages, I compared the "want ads" for male labor from three different years. See *Los Angeles Times*, September 4, 1910; *Los Angeles Times*, September 4, 1911; and *Los Angeles Times*, September 8, 1912.
30. *IDNR* (1898–1907): 9–10.
31. *HDAR* (1911): 6, 31.
32. *IDNR* (1911–1912): 12.
33. Elizabeth Baurhyte was married to William Baurhyte, an executive officer of the Los Angeles Gas and Electric Company. Baurhyte was a member of the Ebell and Friday Morning Club and president of the Los Angeles District of the California Federation of Women's Clubs from 1912 to 1913. William A. Spalding, *History of Los Angeles*, vol. 2 (Los Angeles: J. R. Finnell and Sons, 1931), 112–114; Rockwell D. Hunt, *California and Californians*, vol. 4 (Chicago: Lewis, 1926), 25–26. The Florence Crittenton Home was a local chapter of a national organization. See Katherine G. Aiken, *Harnessing the Power of Motherhood: The National Crittenton Mission,*

1883–1925 (Knoxville: University of Tennessee Press, 1998); Peggy Pascoe, *Relations of Rescue: The Search for Female Moral Authority in the American West, 1874–1939* (New York: Oxford University Press, 1990); Otto Wilson, *Fifty Years' Work with Girls, 1883–1933: A Story of the Florence Crittenton Homes* (Alexandria, Va.: National Florence Crittenton Mission, 1933).

34. Otto Wilson, *Fifty Years' Work with Girls*, 1; "Our Maternity Cottage," Box 84, Folder 3, Caroline Severance Collection, Huntington Library.
35. In 1910, the Los Angeles County Medical Association adopted a fee bill setting the price that physicians should charge a patient for an uncomplicated labor from $25 to $150. More difficult births ranged from $50 to $500 and a caesarean section could cost anywhere from $250 to $2,500. See *State Directory of Physicians and Surgeons* (1916), 129.
36. Litoff, *American Midwives*, 128–129.
37. Municipal Charities Commission, *Annual Reports of the Municipal Charities Commission of the City of Los Angeles, California* (1914–1924).
38. *IDNR* (1910–1911): 7.
39. Gertrude Jacinta Fraser, *African American Midwifery in the South: Dialogues of Birth, Race, and Memory* (Cambridge, Mass.: Harvard University Press, 1998); Margaret Charles Smith, *Listen to Me Good: The Life Story of an Alabama Midwife* (Columbus, Ohio: Ohio State University Press, 1996); Laural Thatcher Ulrich, *A Midwife's Tale: The Life of Martha Ballard Based on Her Diary, 1785–1812* (New York: Alfred A. Knopf, 1990); Linda V. Walsh, "Midwives as Wives and Mothers: Urban Midwives in the Early Twentieth Century," *Nursing History Review* 2 (1994): 51–65.
40. After 1910, the health department's annual report listed an aggregate number of permits issued, and it was always greater than the numbers listed in the city directory. The United States Census provides another numerical glimpse. Although categorized with nurses, in 1900, census takers recorded 489. When the two categories were split in 1920, the census classified only 19 women as midwives.
41. I was able to determine the ethnic origin of 84 out of the 105 names listed in the city directory using Patrick Hanks and Flavia Hodges, *A Dictionary of Surnames* (New York: Oxford University Press, 1988), and Elsdon C. Smith, *New Dictionary of American Family Names* (New York: Harper and Row, 1973).
42. See 1900, 1910, and 1920, United States Census Manuscript; Los Angeles City Directories, 1887–1927. Lisa See, *On Golden Mountain: The One-Hundred-Year Odyssey of My Chinese-American Family* (New York: Vintage Books, 1995): 65, 80.
43. See 1900 and 1910 United States Census Manuscript; *Los Angeles City Directories*, 1887–1915.
44. See 1900 United States Census Manuscript; *Los Angeles City Directories*, 1887–1908.
45. For Louisa Claussen, see *Los Angeles City Directories*, 1895–1911. For Wiebecke Kruse, see *Los Angeles City Directories*, 1891–1915. For Emma Bergstedt, see *Los Angeles City Directories*, 1890–1920.
46. Smith was born in West Virginia in 1850 and she married her second husband, James Smith, the same year that she opened her institution. Their household also included two daughters, one from Smith's previous marriage and one they had adopted in 1888. Although her husband worked steadily as a carpenter, Smith owned the property.
47. Advertisement in the *Los Angeles City Directory*, 1893.

48. "Report of Obstetrical Cases," *Southern California Practitioner* 6, no. 11 (1891): 505–509.
49. Board of Health Minutes, December 2, 1908, and March 17, 1909, LACA.
50. "Quadruplets Attract Women," *Los Angeles Examiner*, January 23, 1910.
51. "Dr. Pratt Declares Wilson Quadruplets Hoax," *Los Angeles Examiner*, January 24, 1910.
52. "I Borrowed 4 Babes for Mrs. Wilson Says Mrs. Smith," *Los Angeles Examiner*, January 25, 1910.
53. "Wilson Quadruplets in New Home. Wait Identification," *Los Angeles Examiner*, January 27, 1910; "Court Seizes Hoax Quadruplets from Pseudo Mother," *Los Angeles Examiner*, January 28, 1910; "Baby Hoax Witness Is Menaced," *Los Angeles Examiner*, May 23, 1910; "Mrs. Wilson Gets Hoax Babies," *Los Angeles Examiner*, June 29, 1910. "Child Stealing Story Repeated," *Los Angeles Times*, June 7, 1910; "Quadruplet Case," *Los Angeles Times*, June 8, 1910; "Stolidly Hears Words," *Los Angeles Times*, June 10, 1910.
55. "Condemns Mrs. Smith," *Los Angeles Times*, June 29, 1910.
56. "Aged Child Stealer Saved from Prison," *Los Angeles Examiner*, June 30, 1910.
57. *IDNR* (1908–1910): 7.
58. *HDAR* (1915): 99. This figure is based on the calendar year rather than the health department's fiscal year-end review.
59. Census data indicates that the percentage of southern and eastern Europeans jumped from 8 percent of all foreign-born immigrants residing in Los Angeles in 1900 to 20 percent in 1910 and 24 percent in 1920. In addition, the percentage of Japanese in the city increased from less than 1 percent to 6 percent during this same time period. See Fogelson, *Fragmented Metropolis*, 76.
60. City Council Minutes, vol. 150, page 790 (1924), LACA. City Archives Petition No. 7478 (1924), LACA.
61. Lyle G. McNeile was born in Iowa in 1885. He received his schooling in New York but obtained his medical degree from the University of California, Southern Branch (formerly the College of Medicine), in 1910, where he met his future wife, Olga Murray. Olga McNeile was born in Chicago in 1893. Like her husband, she became a specialist in gynecology and obstetrics. See "Grades for 1908–09 session-junior class," in Box 2, Folder 4, Los Angeles Medical Department Collection, UCLA University Archives; *Who's Who in California: A Biographical Dictionary* (1928–1929), 613. It is possible that McNeile might have been influenced by the ideas of Joseph De Lee. Upon graduation, Lyle McNeile returned to New York to pursue his post-graduate studies at the Sloane Hospital for Women. He then became a resident physician at the Chicago Lying-In Hospital, which was headed by De Lee. De Lee was vehement about eliminating the practice of midwifery and remained firmly committed to hospital births. A few months before Los Angeles established its program, however, De Lee published an article in which he suggested that voluntary associations and municipalities hire obstetricians to enter people's homes as a temporary alternative. Joseph B. De Lee, "Progress toward Ideal Obstetrics," *Transactions of the American Association for the Study and Prevention of Infant Mortality* 6 (1915): 114–123.
62. "Babies of Poor Get a Chance," *Los Angeles Times*, June 14, 1914.
63. *HDAR* (1920): 32. He was probably correct. New York, the most often credited leader in public health innovation, did not create its Maternity Center Association until 1918. Furthermore, it provided only prenatal care and relied on the Henry Street

Nursing settlement to provide postpartum care. See Mazyck P. Ravenel, *A Half Century of Public Health* (New York: American Public Health Association, 1921), 310. The quote came after a month-long tour McNeile conducted in the winter of 1919 to see other facilities. See City Archives Petition No. 2775 (1919); City Council Minutes, vol. 116, page 70 (1919), LACA.

64. *HDAR* (1925): 44–45. "Babies of Poor Get a Chance," *Los Angeles Times*, June 14, 1914.
65. J. J. Jessup, *Annexation Map and Digest of City Charters* (Los Angeles: Department of Public Works, 1931).
66. *HDAR* (1918): 30–31.
67. *HDAR* (1918): 27. Ruth Janetta Temple and Tahi Lani Mottl, *Interview with Ruth Janetta Temple: June 12, 1978.* Black Women Oral History Project. ([Cambridge, Mass.]: Schlesinger Library, Radcliffe College, 1980), 13.
68. *HDAR* (1916): 8–9.
69. *HDAR* (1912): 72.
70. *HDAR* (1917): 37.
71. Regarding McNeile's statistics and expectations see *HDAR* (1916): 7, 11; *HDAR* (1917): 37; *HDAR* (1925): 44.
72. City Council Minutes, vol. 150, page 790 (1924), LACA. City Archives Petition No. 7478 (1924), LACA.
73. City Council Minutes, vol. 118, page 674 (1920); City Council Minutes, vol. 126, page 766 (1922); City Council Minutes, vol. 150, page 790 (1924); LACA. City Archives Petition No. 7478 (1924), LACA.
74. *HDAR* (1917): 37.
75. California Statutes (1917), chapter 81.
76. City Archives Petition No. 2902 (1919), LACA.
77. *HDAR* (1917): 40; *HDAR* (1918): 30.
78. The source for this midwife's testimony comes from the California State Archives, Professional and Vocational Standards: Deceased Physician Files. These records include obituaries and applications for certification. In using these materials I am restricted from revealing specific individual identities.
79. *HDAR* (1920): 30.
80. These women's stories come from the California State Archives, Professional and Vocational Standards: Deceased Physician Files. See note 78.
81. *HDAR* (1915): 99. Sirch noted that the next largest groups, in order, were Italian, Mexican, American, and Austrian. For a comparison of the prevalence of Japanese midwives in the Far West, see Susan L. Smith, "The 'Midwife Problem' in the Far West: Japanese Midwives in Hawaii and Washington," in Steven Totosy de Zepetnek and Jennifer W. Jay, eds., *East Asia Cultural Historical Perspectives* (Alberta, Canada: University of Alberta, Research Institute for Comparative Literature and Cross-Cultural Studies, 1997), 163–171.
82. Albert Camarillo has estimated the Japanese population in 1910 at four thousand. Camarillo, *Chicanos in a Changing Society*. See also Valerie Matsumoto, "Japanese American Women and the Creation of Urban Nisei Culture in the 1930s," in Valerie J. Matsumoto and Blake Allmendinger, eds., *Over the Edge: Remapping the American West* (Berkeley: University of California Press, 1999), 292.
83. Smith, *Japanese American Midwives*, chapter 1. See also Mary W. Standlee, *The Great Pulse: Japanese Midwifery and Obstetrics through the Ages* (Rutland, VT: Charles E. Tuttle, 1959), 37–38.

84. Between 1900 and 1910, the Italian population in Los Angeles grew from 763 to 3,802 and doubled in the next decade to 7,931. See Bureau of the Census, *Abstract of the Thirteenth Census: Foreign Born Population by Country of Birth in Cities Having 250,000 Inhabitants or More: 1910 and 1900* (Washington, D.C.: GPO, 1910); Bureau of the Census, *Abstract of the Fourteenth Census: Foreign Born Population by Country of Birth in Cities Having 100,000 Inhabitants or More: 1910 and 1900* (Washington, D.C.: GPO, 1920).
85. Regarding midwifery training in Italy, see Vecchio, *Merchants, Midwives, and Laboring Women*, chapter 4.
86. Unfortunately, the division did not break these numbers down by race, class, and ethnicity.
87. City Council Minutes, vol. 241, page 411 (1933), LACA ; City Council Minutes, vol. 242, page 514 (1933), LACA. I am indebted to Natalia Molina for drawing my attention to these records.
88. City Council Minutes, vol. 240, page 302 (1933), LACA. City Archives Petition No. 3161 (1933), LACA.
89. City Archives Petition No. 3741 (1933), LACA.
90. City Council Minutes, vol. 242, page 368 (1933), LACA.
91. City Archives Petition No. 4946 (1933), LACA.
92. City Archives Petition No. 4662 (1933), LACA. See also City Archives Petition No. 4895 (1933), LACA; City Council Minutes, vol. 240, page 762 (1933), LACA.
93. *HDAR* (1933): 11.
94. City Council Minutes, vol. 242, page 368 (1933), LACA.

Chapter 5: The Challenge of Constructing Venereal Disease Programs

1. *HDAR* (1919): 50.
2. Christopher Capozzola, "The Only Badge Needed Is Your Patriotic Fervor: Vigilance, Coercion, and the Law in World War I America," *Journal of American History* 88(4) (2002): 1354–1382.
3. Estelle B. Freedman, *Their Sisters' Keepers: Women's Prison Reform in America, 1830–1930* (Ann Arbor: University of Michigan Press, 1981); Timothy J. Gilfoyle, *A Pickpocket's Tale: The Underworld of Nineteenth-Century New York* (New York: W. W. Norton, 2006).
4. David J. Pivar, *Purity and Hygiene: Women, Prostitution, and the "American Plan," 1900–1930* (Westport, Conn.: Greenwood, 2002), 109–111.
5. According to the health department's statistics, 37.7 percent of all men examined at the Central Jail had some form of venereal disease as compared to 64.4 percent of all the women examined. *HDAR* (1919): 45.
6. Arthur M. Rogers (1869–1945) became the clinic's second supervisor in 1919 and remained in charge of the city's venereal disease division through the 1930s. His younger brother, Alfred R. Rogers (1871–1939), was the first supervisor. Both were born in Iowa, where they received their medical training, and moved to Los Angeles in the 1910s. See *HDAR* (1919): 44–45; Minutes, Los Angeles Urological Association (1918–1947), Huntington Library; "Funeral Friday for Dr. Rogers," *Los Angeles Times*, November 29, 1939. "Dr. A. M. Rogers Taken by Death," *Los Angeles Times*, October 22, 1945.
7. Allan M. Brandt, *No Magic Bullet: A Social History of Venereal Diseases in the United States since 1880* (New York: Oxford University Press, 1987), especially chapters 2 and 3; Nancy K. Bristow, *Making Men Moral: Social Engineering during*

the Great War (New York: New York University Press, 1996); Mark Thomas Connelly, *The Response to Prostitution in the Progressive Era* (Chapel Hill: University of North Carolina Press, 1980); Barbara Meil Hobson, *Uneasy Virtue: The Politics of Prostitution and the American Reform Tradition* (New York: Basic Books, 1987), chapter 7; Adam Hodges, "'Enemy Aliens' and 'Silk Stocking Girls': The Class Politics of Internment in the Drive for Urban Order during World War I," *Journal of the Gilded Age and Progressive Era* 6, no. 4 (2007): 431–458; David J. Pivar, "Cleansing the Nation: The War on Prostitution, 1917–21," *Prologue*, Spring 1980, 29–40; Claude Quétel, *The History of Syphilis*, trans. Judith Braddock and Brian Pike (Baltimore: Johns Hopkins University Press, 1990), 188–189 and 228–233; Nancy Moore Rockafellar, "Making the World Safe for the Soldiers of Democracy: Patriotism, Public Health, and Venereal Disease Control on the West Coast, 1910–1919" (Ph.D. diss., University of Washington, 1990).

8. Regarding working-class women's leisure activities that caused middle-class reformers angst, see Kathy Peiss, *Cheap Amusements: Working Women and Leisure in Turn-of-the-Century New York* (Philadelphia: Temple University Press, 1986), especially chapter 7. Regarding reformers and working-class parents' efforts to respond to these popular amusements by policing female juvenile behavior, see Appier, *Policing Women*; Freedman, *Maternal Justice*; and Odem, *Delinquent Daughters*.

9. Regarding changing social constructions and geographies of prostitution, see Patricia Cline Cohen, *The Murder of Helen Jewitt* (New York: Vintage Press, 1999); Gilfoyle, *City of Eros*; Ruth Rosen, *The Lost Sisterhood: Prostitution in America, 1900–1918* (Baltimore: John Hopkins University Press, 1982); Mark Wild, "Red Light Kaleidoscope: Prostitution and Ethnoracial Relations in Los Angeles, 1880–1940," *Journal of Urban History* 28, no. 6 (2002): 720–742.

10. F. D. Bullard, "Acute Gonorrhea as Treated by Dr. Ernst Finger of Vienna," *Southern California Practitioner* 4, no. 9 (1889): 398.

11. This amended Section 2979a of the California political code.

12. California State Board of Health, *Twenty-fifth Biennial Report of the State Board of Health of California* (1916–1918), 175.

13. *HDAR* (1919): 19.

14. According to Gerald Woods, the 1902 charter reform banning vice within city limits did not work because the police took payoffs to protect these lucrative businesses. Joseph Gerald Woods, "The Progressives and the Police: Urban Reform and the Professionalization of the Los Angeles Police" (Ph.D. diss., University of California, Los Angeles, 1973), 25–27.

15. This action did not go uncontested. In 1914, a group of landlords formed the Los Angeles Rooming-House and Apartment-House Keepers' Association. They objected to the physical damage policemen inflicted upon their property in carrying out the city's anti-vice measures. "Organization to 'Protect' Hotels," *Los Angeles Times*, August 29, 1914.

16. Christman, "The Best Laid Plans," chapter 3. See also Franklin Hichborn, "The Anti-Vice Movement in California, I. Suppression," *Social Hygiene* 6 (1920): 219–220; "California Women and the Vice Situation," *Survey*, May 3, 1913, 162.

17. Friday Morning Club Scrapbook, vol. 1, page 15, Huntington Library.

18. "Morals Issue Splits Clubs," *Los Angeles Times*, January 24, 1917.

19. *HDAR* (1914): 39.

20. Suzanne Poirier, *Chicago's War on Syphilis, 1937–1940: The Times, The Trib, and the Clap Doctor* (Urbana: University of Illinois Press, 1995), 5. As Allan Brandt and

Mark Thomas Connelly have both pointed out, rates were contentious because very few cities and states collected statistics on these diseases. See Brandt, *Magic Bullet*, 12–13; Connelly, *The Response to Prostitution*, 20–22.

21. The ordinance was passed on June 30, 1914. See *HDMR* (April–May 1918): 6–7; Editorial, "Physical Examination of Prostitutes," *Southern California Practitioner* 29, no. 6 (1914): 201–202.
22. Olga McNeile, "The Results of an Examination for the Juvenile Court," *Southern California Practitioner* 28, no. 1 (1913): 52. The reason for the difference in timing between investigating young men and women's bodies is undocumented. In general, this action followed a general increase in female reformers' attempts to police young women in Los Angeles. Odem, *Delinquent Daughters*, 110. Most likely, McNeile was the first female physician to be appointed to the court, and contemporary rules of decorum would have dictated that girls not be subjected to an exam by a male physician.
23. McNeile, "The Results of an Examination," 52–55. Given the long-standing public association of prostitution with venereal disease, McNeile's belief that young women's sexual transgressions would lead to the acquisition of syphilis or gonorrhea is unsurprising. See Linda E. Merians, *The Secret Malady: Venereal Disease in the Eighteenth Century: Britain and France* (Lexington: University Press of Kentucky, 1996); Quetel, *History of Syphilis*, chapter 9; Mary Spongberg, *Feminizing Venereal Disease: The Body of the Prostitute in Nineteenth-Century Medical Discourse* (New York: New York University Press, 1997).
24. I have not found any statistical or anecdotal information in the annual reports of the health or police department.
25. It is also possible that San Francisco's attempt at creating a clinic to treat prostitutes made city officials in Los Angeles wary. Regarding San Francisco, see George E. Malsbary, "The Municipal Clinic of San Francisco," *Southern California Practitioner* 28, no. 5 (1913): 159–167. Rockafellar, "Making the World Safe," 112–124.
26. *HDAR* (1914): 39. Unfortunately for my purposes, the 1915 and 1916 reports do not break down the numbers by sex.
27. Los Angeles Board of Health Commissioners, "Syphilis and Gonorrhea: What the City Health Department Is Doing" (1937), 1.
28. *HDAR* (1918): 16.
29. Ibid. See also *HDMR* (March–April 1918): 5–7.
30. *HDAR* (1917): 19.
31. Los Angeles was unusual in its use of Salvarsan. According to historian Allan M. Brandt, by 1915 many physicians had switched to using Neosalvarsan, which was less deadly but also less effective. See Brandt, *Magic Bullet*, 41. Health department records from Los Angeles do not indicate why they made this choice.
32. Editorial, "Ehrlich's '606' Specific for Syphilis," *Southern California Practitioner* 25, no. 10 (1910): 451.
33. Editorial, "Journal A.M.A.," *Southern California Practitioner* 25, no. 10 (1910): 450.
34. Miscellaneous, "Three New Deaths from Salvarsan," *Southern California Practitioner* 27, no. 1 (1912): 189–190. (reprinted from *JAMA*).
35. Editorial, "Salvarsan Therapy—Its Present Status," *Southern California Practitioner* 27, no. 1 (1912): 24–25.
36. *HDAR* (1919): 47.
37. Ibid., 48.
38. *HDAR* (1918): 48.

39. Ibid., 41; *HDAR* (1919): 49.
40. *HDAR* (1918): 41.
41. *HDAR* (1917): 25.
42. *HDMR* (March–April 1918): 5–7. When the women's division was established, it did not suffer the same problems of staffing. State law obliged local officials to employ a female physician in cases where the patient demanded one; Los Angeles's officials viewed it as a necessity for all cases involving a woman. Consequently, the city opened up opportunities for female physicians at a time when they began to face greater obstacles to maintaining a presence within the male-dominated medical profession. Four different female physicians worked in the women's venereal disease division during this time period: Etta C. Jeancon, Mona Bettin, Hannah Betty, and Emily Bolcom.
43. Alfred Rogers also saw another advantage to employing a physician. Building on the idea of visiting nursing, Rogers instructed his assistant to use his spare time to follow up on patients who resisted returning to the clinic. *HDMR* (February–March 1918): 5–7.
44. In 1919, the army estimated that in Los Angeles for every hundred new recruits, three showed up with a venereal disease. Editorial, "The Percentage of Venereal Diseases among Approximately the Second Million Drafted Men—By Cities," *Southern California Practitioner* 34, no. 8 (1919): 122–123.
45. Brandt, *No Magic Bullet*, 77.
46. Paul B. Johnson, "Social Hygiene and the War," *Social Hygiene* 4 (1918): 105. *The Twenty-Fifth Biennial Report of the State Board of Health of California for the Fiscal Years from July 1, 1916, to June 30, 1918* (California State Printing Office, Sacramento, 1918), 172. According to the Morals Efficiency Association, the state allocated $60,000 toward Los Angeles's venereal disease programs. See Morals Efficiency Association, "Measures for the Prevention of Venereal Diseases in Soldiers and Sailors Stationed in California," Box 73, Folder 68, John Randolph Haynes Collection, Charles E. Young Research Library, Department of Special Collections, University of California, Los Angeles.
47. Rockafellar, "Making the World Safe," chapter 5.
48. *HDMR* (February 1918): 5–8.
49. Editorial, "Federal Trade Commission Acts on Salvarsan Patent," *Southern California Practitioner* 32, no. 12 (1917): 192–193.
50. *HDAR* (1918): 17 and 46; *HDAR* (1919): 44–45.
51. City Archives Petition No. 976 (1918), LACA.
52. *HDAR* (1920): 18.
53. Los Angeles City Police Department, *Annual Report of the Police Department of the City of Los Angeles* (1918), 6.
54. War Department Commission on Training Camp Activities, "What Some Communities of the West and Southwest Have Done for the Protection of the Soldiers and Sailors," October 7, 1917, Box 73, Folder 6, John Randolph Haynes Collection, Charles E. Young Research Library, Department of Special Collections, University of California, Los Angeles.
55. Frank R. Keefer, *Military Hygiene and Sanitation* (Philadelphia: W. B. Saunders, 1918), 282.
56. I believe the health department named this structure Los Feliz Hospital because it was located at 1450 Los Feliz Road. The city has since renamed the road Riverside Drive. Originally built by the Board of Education to serve as a juvenile detention

home, the building had more recently served as a small rehabilitation center for alcoholics.
57. Brandt, *No Magic Bullet*, 84–92; Bristow, *Making Men Moral*, 119–136; *Pivar, Purity and Hygiene*, 210–211.
58. Paul B. Johnson, "Social Hygiene and the War," *Social Hygiene* 4 (1918): 105.
59. The *Los Angeles Times* reported that this made Los Angeles the first city in the nation to open this kind of hospital; however, I have been unable to verify this claim. "New Hospital Born of War," *Los Angeles Times*, January 27, 1918.
60. HDMR (May–June 1918): 8.
61. Rose Baruch was married to Berthold Baruch. In 1913, his estate was estimated at $15,000, which would be approximately $315,000 in 2006. See James Edward Condon, *Southern California Blue Book of Money: Taxpayers Assessed on $5,000 and Upwards* (1913.) Baruch's interest in social hygiene appears to have begun in the mid-1910s, when she was in her early fifties. In reporting Baruch's election as treasurer for the Friday Morning Club, an unidentified newspaper clipping from July 1, 1916, stated that Baruch "has a little hobby, which she hopes will some day materialize into something more than a hobby. She is a firm believer in the instruction of sex hygiene, but she does not believe it should be introduced in the grammar grades." Friday Morning Club Scrapbook, vol 4, page 92, Huntington Library. For biographical information, see *Who's Who in California (1928–29)* (San Francisco: Who's Who Publishing, n.d.), 81. See also "School Immorality Charges Fall Flat," *Los Angeles Times*, December 4, 1914.
62. *HDAR* (1918): 47.
63. See Los Angeles City Police Department, *Annual Report of the Police Department of the City of Los Angeles* (1925–1929), for breakdowns by race and crimes.
64. *HDAR* (1918): 47.
65. Ibid.
66. Friday Morning Club Scrapbook, (vol. 1, page 15), Huntington Library.
67. *HDMR* (May–June 1918): 8.
68. Ibid.
69. "Five WMEN [sic] Break Out of Hospital," *Los Angeles Times*, June 5, 1919; "Was She Kidnapped?" *Los Angeles Times*, September 28, 1921; "Masculine Ways Flees Hospital," *Los Angeles Times*, April 12, 1927.
70. Adam J. Hodges, "Protecting Soldiers, Policing Working-Class Women: Combating Venereal Disease in Portland, Oregon during World War I," paper presented at the Social Science History Association Annual Conference, Chicago, 2004; Bristow, *Making Men Moral*, 129.
71. Alma Whitaker, "Women's Work, Women's Clubs," *Los Angeles Times*, March 28, 1918; *HDAR* (1918): 47.
72. Susan Craddock, *City of Plagues*, 184.
73. City Archives Petition No. 2338 (1919), LACA
74. *HDAR* (1919): 50.
75. *HDAR* (1932): 47.
76. *HDAR* (1924): 50.
77. *HDAR* (1920): 19.
78. See *In re Barmore*, 174 Cal. 286 (1917); *In re Kenne*, 34 Cal. App. 263 (1917); *In re Hah*, 34 Cal. App. 35 (1917); *In re Smith*, 33 Cal. App. 161 (1917); *In re Wisner*, 32 Cal. App. 637 (1917); *In re Saul*, 32 Cal. App. 531 (1917); *In re McCready*, 179 Cal. 514 (1918); *In re Hittson*, 39 Cal. App. 91 (1918); *In re Dowell*, 36 Cal. App. 587

(1918); In re Schwitalla, 36 Cal. App. 511 (1918). The archival record does not indicate whether it was the women or their lawyers who decided on this legal strategy. Historical studies of prostitution, however, indicate that prostitutes' previous experiences with the criminal justice system would have led them to recognize the application of this public health measure as an anomaly. See Rosen, *The Lost Sisterhood*; Josie Washburn, *The Underworld Sewer: A Prostitute Reflects on Life in the Trade, 1871–1909* (Lincoln: University of Nebraska Press, 1997).

79. See *In re Brodie*, 33 Cal. App. 808 (1918); *In re Johnson*, 36 Cal. App. 319 (1918).
80. Under the auspices of the Commission on Training Camp Activities (CTCA), the federal government adopted a policy of quarantine. However, many leading female reformers engaged in CTCA activities believed that this was an inappropriate and unjust policy because it treated men and women differently, placed the blame on women, and lacked any policy for rehabilitation. See Appier, *Policing Women*, 43–45; Odem, *Delinquent Daughters*, 124–126; David J. Pivar, "Cleansing the Nation: The War on Prostitution, 1917–21," *Prologue*, Spring 1980. The Chamberlain-Kahn Act did not expire until 1923. Consequently, it continued to impact postwar public health policies.
81. *HDAR* (1919): 50–51.
82. Letter from Campbell to Dr. F. F. Gundrum, Acting Secretary of the State Board of Health, dated June 11, 1918, Public Health Folder 3204-142, California State Archives (hereafter CSA).
83. The Los Angeles County health commissioner, J. L. Pomeroy, had asked a similar question a few months before this meeting. See Letter from Campbell to Dr. Wilfred H. Kellogg, Secretary of the State Board of Health, dated April 22, 1918, CSA Public Health Folder 3204-142.
84. See *In re Johnson*, 40 Cal. App. 242 (1919), and Criminal no. 654, California Appellate Court Records, CSA. The decision published Grace Johnston's name as Johnson, but the court records indicate that the former was correct.
85. The most famous contemporary case of a prisoner making use of science to contest her detention was Mary Mallon. See Judith Walzer Leavitt, *Typhoid Mary: Captive to the Public's Health* (Boston: Beacon Press, 1996), 32–33, 73–74.
86. Archival sources do not reveal why Paul Wadsworth Schenck took this case or why he would take a similar case for Mrs. A. Arata in 1921. He used habeas corpus for a male client who was accused of murder in early 1918. See *People v. Denman*, 179 Cal. App. 497 (1918). Before his life was cut short by a heart attack at the age of fifty eight, Schenck was a well-known defense attorney. See Willoughby Rodman, *History of the Bench and Bar of Southern California* (Los Angeles: William J. Porter, 1909); *Who's Who in the Pacific Southwest* (Los Angeles: Times-Mirror Printing and Binding House, 1913); John Steven McGroarty, *Los Angeles from the Mountains to the Sea* (Chicago: American Historical Society, 1921); William A. Spalding, History of Los Angeles (Los Angeles: J. R. Finnell and Sons, 1931); *Los Angeles Times*, December 2, 1932; *Los Angeles Times*, December 6, 1932.
87. *In re Milstead*, 44 Cal. App. 239 (1919), and Criminal no. 685, California Appellate Court Records, CSA, see also "Hits Blow at Lodging Law," *Los Angeles Times*, November 13, 1919.
88. *In re Arata*, 52 Cal. App. 380 (1921), and Criminal no. 790, California Appellate Court Records, CSA.
89. *In Re Dayton*, 52 Cal. App. 635 1921, and Criminal no. 797, California Appellate Court Records, CSA; see also "Blood Test Ruling Not Enforcible," *Los Angeles Times*, April 20, 1921.

90. See *In re Clemente*, 61 Cal. App. 666 (1923), and Criminal no. 987, California Appellate Court Records, CSA; and *In re King*, 128 Cal. App. 27 (1932), and Criminal no. 2294, California Appellate Court Records, CSA.
91. "Nine Los Feliz Inmates Escape," *Los Angeles Times*, May 22, 1921.
92. "City Hospital is Condemned," *Los Angeles Times*, October 29, 1924.
93. City Council Minutes, vol. 204, page 124 (1929), LACA.
94. "Hospital Opening Asked," *Los Angeles Times*, October 17, 1934.
95. Bess M. Wilson, "Mrs. Barton Urges Aid for Neglected Women," *Los Angeles Times*, September 9, 1941.

Conclusion

1. *HDAR* (1932): 8.
2. Ibid., 10.

Index

Italicized page numbers refer to figures.

Acheson, Kathleen, 21
Adams, Ethel, 151–152
Addams, Jane, 6–8, 21, 157
adobes, 47–48, 50, 65, 113, 172n16
adoption, 117–118, 184n46
African Americans, 50, 63, 113, 123, 145, 149, 153, 174n63
alcoholism, 132, 145, 190–191n56
Alembic Club, 101
Alexander, George, 91–92, 96, 120
Alpine Dairy Company, 82–84, 177n23
Anti-Tuberculosis League, 34
apartment houses, 53, 72, 74, 136, 188n15. *See also* tenements
Arata, Mrs. A., 152–153, 192n86
Armstrong, Milton W., 73, 175n112
Armstrong, Sarah J., 73, 175n112
arsenic, 135, 139
Arsphenamine, 143
assimilation, 106, 124, 130, 159

Baldwin, Marie, 154
Bartlett, Dana, 35, 54–55, 60, 71
Barton, Minnie, 155
Baruch, Rose, 145, 191n61
Bason, Manly, 98
Baurhyte, Elizabeth, 114, 183–184n33
Bellamy, Edward, 3
Bergstedt, Emma, 115–117
Bergstrom, George E., 59–60, 173n49
Berryman, Valentine, 153–154
Bethlehem Institute, 34–35, 54–56, 166n27
Bettin, Mona, 140, 143, 146–148, 150–151, 190n42
Bingham, Mary, 10
birth registration, 107, 124
boardinghouses, 15, 40, 50, 116
Bouton, Edward, 15–17
bovine tuberculosis, 90–93, 97–98, 100, 102, 179n69

Bristow, Nancy, 147
Brownson House, 35, 54, 56, 123, 166n27
Bullard, Rose, 136, 146
Bundy, Augusta, 115–116
Bureau of District Nursing, 38, 41, 123
Bureau of Housing, 73–76
Bureau of Municipal Nursing, 41–43, 73, 170n106
Bureau of Social Hygiene, 142

California Appellate Court, 149–154
California Federation of Women's Clubs, 63–64, 92, 102–103, 183–184n33
California State Board of Health, 116, 127, 135, 142, 144, 149
California State Board of Medical Examiners, 117, 127
Campbell, Kemper B., 149–151
carfare, 20, 42, 123, 168n36
Carver, S.W.A., 95
Catholics, 5, 35, 130, 166n27
Catholic Woman's Club, 130
censuses: and housing reform, 45–46, 173n49; and midwifery/maternity programs, 107, 112, 115–117, 121, 182n6, 183n21, 184n40, 185n59, 187n84; and milk reform, 79, 88; and public health nursing, 20–21, 27–28
certified milk, 85–86, 92, 99, 178n40
Chamberlain-Kahn Act (July 1918), 142, 149, 192n80
charities, 5, 11–14, 24, 40
Charities and Commons, 57, 66
Chavez, Oscar, 17
Chicago, 2, 6–7, 12, 54, 185n61; and milk reform, 86, 93–94, 99
childbirth, 1, 7–9, 104–131, *105*, 159, 182nn1,2; and housing reform, 67–68, 72; and public health nursing, 30–32; and venereal disease programs, 136. *See also* midwifery
Children's Bureau, 85, 97
Children's Hospital Society, 130

195

Chinese immigrants, 4, 49–50, 63, 70, 116, 174n63
class-based factors, 3, 9, 24, 106; and housing reform, 50, 72, 171n2; and milk reform, 78–79, 88, 95–96, 181n119. *See also* middle-class standards; working classes
Claussen, Louisa, 110, 115–117
clubwomen, 5–6, 157; and housing reform, 44, 46, 53–54, 67–69, 172n34; and midwifery/maternity programs, 183–184n33; and milk reform, 7, 86–92, 94, 102; and public health nursing, 21, 42, 170n106; and venereal disease programs, 136–137, 145–147, 155, 191n61. *See also names of clubs and clubwomen*
Coffey, Titian, 59–60, 63–64, 67–68, 71, 173n49
Cole, George L., 120
college alumnae, 7, 21–22, 169n48
College of Medicine, 33–35, 112, 173n49, 185n61
Collegiate Alumni Association of Los Angeles, 7, 22, 165nn22,23
Collier, Jennie E., 6
Colliver, J. A., 138
Commission of Instructive District Nursing, 38–40
Commission on Training Camp Activities (CTCA), 147, 192n80
Conference of Social Workers (May 1912), 113
Congregationalists, 34, 54–55, 166n27
Connelly, Mark Thomas, 188–189n20
contagious diseases, 5; and housing reform, 50–51, 63, 68; and public health nursing, 18, 28, 35, 40; and venereal disease programs, 135, 139, 146. *See also* epidemics; *specific contagious diseases*
Conway, E. A., 153
Council of Catholic Women, 130
Council of Jewish Women, 130, 166n27
Crescent Creamery, 82, 95

dairy industry, 8, 77–86, 88–96, 98–100, 102, 176nn7,9, 177n23, 178n40, 180n83
Dairymen's Union, 82

Day, William Horace, 59, 173n49
Dayton, Betty, 153–154
Decker, C. W., 33, 156
DeForest, Robert W., 62
De Lee, Joseph, 185n61
Dillon, Frank, 151–152
diphtheria, 5, 19, 28–30, 49, 56, 61, 90–91, 168n29
dispensaries, 33–35, 105, 122–125
District Nursing Program (LACSA). *See* Bureau of District Nursing
Division of Obstetrics (Los Angeles City Health Dept.), 104, 121–127, 130–131, 185n61, 185–186n63, 187n86

Eades, Jessie, 151–152
Ebell Club, 53, 67–68, 94, 96, 130, 183–184n33
Edson, Katherine Philips, 74, 77–78, 85–90, 92–99, 101–103, 178n43, 182n129
Ehrlich, Paul, 135, 139, 158
Eighth Ward, 34–35, 113, 168n31; and housing reform, 46, 50, 52, 56, 67
Electrical Workers Union, 62
El Hogar Felis, 56
Elsing, William T., 47–48, 62
England. *See* Great Britain
Engleman, Sadie, 118–120
epidemics, 2, 4–5, 8, 26, 37–40, 52, 57, 90–91
Episcopal Church, 5, 34, 147, 166n27
ethnicity, 9, 159; and housing reform, 45–46, 50, 61–62, 65; and midwifery/maternity programs, 112, 115, 123, 128–131, 182n6, 184n41, 185n59, 186nn81,82; and milk reform, 121; and public health nursing, 15, 19, 24–26; and venereal disease programs, 145. *See also* race factors
European immigrants (eastern/southern), 4–5, 46, 58, 106, 121, 128, 185n59

female inspectors, 10; and housing reform, 44, 47, 66–73, *70,* 75; and milk reform, 103; and public health nursing, 30, 42
female physicians, 123, 145–146, 153, 189n22, 190n42. *See also names of female physicians*

female prisoners, 132–134, 137–138, 143–153, 187n5, 191–192nn78, 192n85
female reformers, 2–9, 156–160, 165n26, 166n29; and housing reform, 46–47, 55, 61, 72–76, 171n5; and midwifery/maternity programs, 106, 111, 113, 130, 156; and milk reform, 78, 84–85; and public health nursing, 10–13, 18, 20, 41, 43; and venereal disease programs, 132, 134–137, 140, 155–156, 188n8, 189n22, 192n80. *See also names of female reformers and organizations*
feminism, 134–135, 165n26
Fette, M. M., 46
Flexner, Abraham, 33
Florence Crittenton Home, 114, 183–184n33
folk medicine/tradition, 24–25. *See also* quackery
Foster, Maude B., 10, 14–16, 18–19, 21, 168nn37–39. *See also* Weston, Maude Foster
Foster, Nancy, 20–21
Franco, Dominga C., 110, 183n21
Franco, Jose, 17–18
French immigrants, 15, 47, 49, 123, 128–129
Friday Morning Club (FMC), 5–7, 165n23; and housing reform, 46, 53, 71; and midwifery/maternity programs, 130, 183–184n33; and milk reform, 86–92, 94, 96; and public health nursing, 21, 170n106; and venereal disease programs, 136, 146, 191n61
Fry, George, 82

Galpin, Kate Tupper, 7
garbage collection, 53–54, 62, 66, 76
Gardner, Placida, 139
Garner, Irene, 146
Geantit, Marie, 47–48
gender factors, 9, 159; and housing reform, 44, 46–47, 57, 59, 65–69, 72–73, 171n2, 173n49; and midwifery/maternity programs, 118, 123; and milk reform, 78, 82–90, 94–97, 100–103, 177n23, 181n119; and public health nursing, 26–27, 40–42, 170n106; and venereal disease programs, 133–135, 137–138, 140, 143–145, 187n5, 188n8, 189nn22,26, 190n42, 192n80. *See also entries beginning with* female
Genito-Urinary Clinic, 134, 138–141, 190nn42,43
Gentleman's Agreement (1907), 128
German immigrants, 15, 49, 115–116, 129
Germany, 99, 132, 143
germ theory, 2, 18–19, 25, 45, 54, 57–58, 81–82, 89, 99
Gibbons, Sherwin, 38
Goins, May, 146
gonorrhea, 132–137, 141–143, 148, 150, 155, 188–189n20, 189n23
Graul, H. S., 82
Great Britain, 11, 27, 46, 68, 88, 107
Great Depression, 9, 130–131, 156
Guiberson, J. W., 102
Gullett, Gayle, 96

habeas corpus, writ of, 132, 148–153, 191–192n78, 192n86
Hahn, Terrill, 152
Halloran, Alice M., 26
Hammond, Samuel F., 21
Harper, Arthur C., 67, 83, 110
Harriman, Job, 96
Hart, George, 92–93, 98–99, 102
Harvey, Louise M., 10
Haverty, Thomas, 60
Haynes, Francis L., 109
Haynes, John Randolph, 71
health inspectors, 10, 12, 30, 35, 40, 42, 49–50, 64, 81. *See also* housing inspectors; milk inspectors
health professionals. *See* medical profession
Hearst, William Randolph, 96
Henry Street Settlement (New York City), 13, 185–186n63
Hill, Octavia, 68, 71
Hodges, Adam, 147
Holohan, James B., 135
home care, 9, 11, 43, 166n7; and midwifery/maternity programs, 104–106, *105,* 111, 114, 122, 124–125, 131, 185n61; and venereal disease programs, 140. *See also* public health nursing
Hood, George, 80–82, 84

hospitals, 1, 5; and midwifery/maternity programs, 104, 109, 112–115, 117–120, 124–125, 183–184n33, 185n61; and public health nursing, 26–27, 29–31, 40, 42, 170n103; and venereal disease programs, 133–134, 137, 140–141, 143–150, *144,* 154–156, 158, 190–191n56, 191n59
Hotchkiss, E. W., 82
Houghton, Arthur D., 62–63
House Court Ordinance, 64–67
house courts, 8, 37, 45, 51, 56–58, 60–72, *70,* 74–76, 171n5
housing commission, 51, 58–76, 172n21
housing inspectors, 44, 47, 59, 62–63, 66–75, *70*
housing reform, 7–8, 44–76, 156, 159, 171nn2,5; and Bureau of Housing, 73–76; and education, 59, 66, 69, 72–73, 75–76; and house courts, 8, 37, 45, 51, 56–58, 60–72, *70,* 74–76, 171n5; and housing commission, 51, 58–76; and Riis, 8, 44–46, 49–54, 60, 66, 69, 74, 76, 172nn21,30
How the Other Half Lives (Riis), 51
Hull House (Chicago), 6–7, 12, 21, 86
Humane Society. *See* Los Angeles Humane Society for Children
hygienic practices, 2, 7, 72, 75, 88; and midwifery/maternity programs, 108–109, 124, 126; and public health nursing, 25–26, 34–35; and venereal disease programs, 134–136. *See also* sanitation

Ihdler, John, 74
immigrants, 1, 3–5, 7, 157, 159; and housing reform, 45–49, 56, 58, 60–63, 67, 69–73, 75–76, 171n5, 174n63; and midwifery/maternity programs, 104–107, *105,* 110–116, 121–131, 182nn1,2, 185n59, 186nn81,82, 187n84; and public health nursing, 10, 19, 24–26, 28–33, 35, 37
infant mortality, 5, 87–89, 91, 97, 103, 107, 111, 124, 131, 182n6
infection: and midwifery/maternity programs, 108; and milk reform, 67, 93, 97–98; and public health nursing, 18, 26, 31, 33–34; and venereal disease programs, 133–134, 137–138, 141–143, 150–152
Instructive District Nursing Association for the City of Los Angeles, 22
International Medical Congress (Washington, 1908), 98
International Women's Congress, 69
interns. *See* medical students
Italian immigrants, 19, 159; and housing reform, 49–50, 56, 70; and midwifery/maternity programs, 107, 113, 123, 128–129, 186n81, 187n84

Japanese immigrants, 4, 35, 159; and midwifery/maternity programs, 107, 115, 128–130, 185n59, 186nn81,82
Jeancon, Etta C., 132–134, 140, 148–149, 190n42
Jewish Benevolent Society, 5
Jews, 5, 28, 35, 113, 130, 166n27
Johnson, C. F., 150
Johnson, Hiram, 102–103, 182n129
Johnston, Grace, 150–151, 153, 192nn84–86
Jonson, May, 146
Journal of the American Medical Association (JAMA), 139–140
juveniles, 21, 137–138, 149, 188n8, 189n22, 190–191n56

Katz, Sherry, 167n23
Kelley, Florence, 8, 86–88, 157
Kemp, Helen M., 148
Kenney, Elizabeth L., 59–60, 173n49
Kenney, Grace, 146
kidnapping trial, 117–120
Koch, Robert, 90–91, 98
Kress, George H., 39–40
Kruse, Wiebcke, 115–117

labor, 8, 86–87, 103, 113, 146, 183n29
labor unions, 55, 62, 82, 96
LACSA. *See* Los Angeles College Settlement Association
landlords, 49, 56–57, 61–62, 65, 68, 70, 73, 75, 188n15
Landmarks Club, 54
Lane, James B., 51

languages, variety of, 26, 35, 67–70, 110, 122, 124, 126–129
La Primavera Club, 21
Lent, Mary E., 43
Liberal Club, 71
lice, 36, 146
Lindley, Walter, 109
Locke, Charles E., 95
Locke, Laura M., 78, 95–97, 100–101, 103
lodging houses/hotels, 38, 44–45, 55, 58, 74–75, 136, 188n15
Longstreth, Sarah, 6
Looking Backward (Bellamy), 3
Los Angeles Board of Education, 145, 147, 190–191n56
Los Angeles Board of Health, 4, 8, 158–159; and housing reform, 47, 49, 58, 63–64, 67–68; and midwifery/maternity programs, 109–110, 116–117, 120–121, 127, 130, 183n22; and milk reform, 80–82, 84, 89–94; and public health nursing, 10, 12–13, 36–41; and venereal disease programs, 135
Los Angeles Board of Social Workers, 145–147
Los Angeles Butter Board of Trade, 83
Los Angeles Citizen, 97
Los Angeles City Council, 158; and housing reform, 62, 64, 67, 72–73, 175n112; and midwifery/maternity programs, 120, 125, 130; and milk reform, 79–81, 89, 91–94, 180n83; and public health nursing, 11–13, 15–18, 20, 38–41, 167n25; and venereal disease programs, 137–138, 147, 154
Los Angeles City Health Department, 7, 9, 156–159; and housing reform, 49–50, 56, 58–60, 65, 72–76; and midwifery/maternity programs, 104, 113, 118, 120–126, 130–131, 182n6, 184n40, 185n58; and milk reform, 81, 84, 92–93, 101, 103; and public health nursing, 10–13, 18–19, 28, 36–37, 40–42, 167n8; and venereal disease programs, 132–133, 137–139, 141–143, 145–146, 148–149, 152–155, 187n5, 189nn24,31, 190–191n56
Los Angeles City Mission Society, 34

Los Angeles College Settlement Association (LACSA), 1, 5–7, 157–158, 165n22; and housing reform, 44–45, 47–51, 54–60, 63, 65, 73, 76, 172nn16,34, 173n49; and midwifery/maternity programs, 111–115, 121, 123–124; and milk reform, 92; and public health nursing, 10–43, 168n37, 169n48
Los Angeles Country Club, 21
Los Angeles County Charities Department, 131
Los Angeles County Hospital, 27, 114, 118–119, 125, 150
Los Angeles County Medical Association, 122, 184n35
Los Angeles County Medical Society, 39, 98
Los Angeles Creamery Company, 83–84
Los Angeles Daily Examiner, 118
Los Angeles District Federation of Women's Clubs, 94
Los Angeles District Parent-Teachers Association, 130
Los Angeles Examiner, 52, 95–96, 99–102, 181n115
Los Angeles Express, 6–7, 63, 181n115
Los Angeles Forum, 130
Los Angeles Herald, 6, 52, 77, 83, 96–97, 101, 181n115
Los Angeles Humane Society for Children, 31, 34, 169n71
Los Angeles League of Women Voters, 130
Los Angeles Municipal Housing Commission (LAMHC), 71
Los Angeles Municipal News, 96
Los Angeles Public Library, 21
Los Angeles Social Hygiene Association, 145
Los Angeles Society of Social Hygiene, 138
Los Angeles Times, 7; and housing reform, 51–57, 62–63, 65, 67, 69–70; and midwifery/maternity programs, 110, 119–120, 122; and milk reform, 81–83, 88, 96, 101, 181n115; and public health nursing, 22, 37–38; and venereal disease programs, 146, 191n59
Los Feliz Hospital, 133–134, 140–141, 143–150, *144,* 154–156, 158, 190–191n56, 191n59
Lummis, Dorothea, 7

Index

Lusk, Robert Martin, 91
lying-in period. *See* postnatal care

MacGowan, Granville, 49–50
Macy, Cordelia E., 112–113
malaria, 48–49
Mann Act (1910), 136
Mason, Helen, 146
maternalism, 3, 7; and midwifery/maternity programs, 118–119; and milk reform, 85, 90, 95, 97, 100, 103; and venereal disease programs, 134
Maternity Division (Los Angeles City Health Dept.), 121
maternity nurses, 104–106, *105,* 111–114, 117, 123–124, 127–128, 130–131, 183n28
mayors, 158–159; and housing reform, 55, 58–59, 63, 67, 73; and midwifery/maternity programs, 110, 120; and milk reform, 82–83, 91–92, 94, 96; and public health nursing, 12, 39, 41. *See also names of mayors*
McAleer, Owen C., 58
McDonald, E. A., 83
McNeile, Lyle G., 121–125, 127, 185n61, 185–186n63
McNeile, Olga, 121, 123, 138, 185n61, 189n22
McRae, Miss, 22
measles, 5, 19, 37–40, 158
Medical Milk Commission, 85, 89
medical profession, 3–4, 8–9, 158–159; and midwifery/maternity programs, 104–105, 111, 121–122, 185n61; and milk reform, 94, 96, 101; and venereal disease programs, 135, 137, 141. *See also* physicians; public health nursing
medical students, 112, 114, 121–125, 141
Melrose, N. M., 65
Merchants and Manufacturers' Association, 54
mercury, 139–140
Mexican immigrants, 4, 159; and housing reform, 48–50, 56, 58, 62–63, 65, 72–73, 75–76, 171n5; and midwifery/maternity programs, 104–106, *105,* 110, 112–113, 115, 123, 127, 182n1, 186n81; and public

health nursing, 19–20, 25–26, 33; and venereal disease programs, 145
Mexican Revolution, 20, 113
microbes, 78, 82, 89, 91–92, 94, 135
middle-class standards, 3, 5–7; and housing reform, 45–46, 51, 59, 63, 75; and midwifery/maternity programs, 106–107, 112, 114, 118; and milk reform, 77, 79, 84–88, 95, 103; and public health nursing, 10, 20, 28; and venereal disease programs, 188n8
midwifery, 24, 104–131, 159, 182n2, 183nn21,22, 184nn40,41; criminalization of, 118–121, 124, 126–127; and kidnapping trial, 117–120; licenses (permits) for, 107, 109–110, 115–118, 121, 124–130, 183nn21,22, 186nn78,80; vs. obstetrics, 33, 104, 108–109, 111–112, 114–115, 117, 122–127, 130–131, 184n35, 185n61, 187n86; ordinance against, 109–110, 115, 120–121, 126; statistics for, 107, 115, 121, 128–129, 184n40, 185nn58,59, 186nn81,82, 187n84
milk adulteration, 80–81, 83, 89
Milk Consumer's League, 95
milk contamination, 87–91, 98–99
milk depots, 88, 92
milk inspectors, 80–84, 89–90, 92–93, 98–99
milk reform, 7–8, 77–103, 158, 176nn7,9; and bovine tuberculosis, 90–93, 97–98, 100, 102, 179n69; and maternalism, 85, 90, 95, 97, 100, 103; and science, 78, 81–82, 85–86, 88–91, 94, 97–99, 101, 103; and transportation of milk, 80, 84, 92–93, 100; and tuberculin ordinance, 77–79, 85, 89, 91–103, 180n83, 181nn115,119; and tuberculin testing, 77–78, 85–86, 90–95, 97–102, 178n43, 179n69. *See also entries beginning with* milk
milk trust, 82–84, 177n23
Milstead, Florence, 151–152
model housing, 68, 71
Mohler, Frank P., 153
Molina, Natalia, 50, 171n5, 182n1
Monks, Sara P., 6

Morals Efficiency Association, 136–137, 190n46
Morris, Edward J., 12
mortality rates, 5, 49, 72, 88, 107, 182n6
Mueller, Anna, 115–116
Municipal League, 51, 54, 58–59, 64–65
Municipal News, 101–102

National Consumers' League, 8, 86
National Housing Association, 74
National Organization of Public Health Nursing (NOPHN), 43, 166nn1,7, 168n36
Neighborhood House Settlement, 122–123, 166n27
Nelson, Anna, 146
Neosalvarsan, 189n31
New Deal, 156
New York City, 6, 8; and housing reform, 44, 46–47, 50–53, 60, 66, 69, 71, 73; and midwifery/maternity programs, 107, 185n61, 185–186n63; and milk reform, 85–86, 88–89, 103; and public health nursing, 12–13, 18, 36
New York Housing Act (1867), 60
New York Tribune, 69
New York University Settlement, 6, 46
Nightingale, Florence, 27
Niles, William, 81
Ninth Ward, 37, 39, 46, 56, 168n31
nurses. *See* public health nursing

obstetrics, 33, 104, 108–109, 111–112, 114–115, 117, 121–127, 130–131, 184n35, 185n61, 187n86
Oliver, Bryon, 81
overcrowding, 48, 50, 52, 56–58, 60, 64, 66, 71

Parrish, George, 75, 155
pasteurization, 85–86, 93–94, 99
Pellissier, Frank F., 83
Perry, Frank, 152
Peters, Lulu H., 102
Peterson, Guy, 81
philanthropists. *See* private funding
physicians, 1, 9, 59, 158; and midwifery/maternity programs, 104–109, 111–112, 114, 118, 120–126, 130, 184n35, 185n61; and milk reform, 77–78, 86, 90–91, 94–95, 97–98, 101–103; and public health nursing, 10, 13, 18, 24–25, 28, 30, 33, 35, 38–41, 168n29, 170n106; and venereal disease programs, 132, 135, 137–142, 149–150, 153, 189nn22,31, 190nn42–43
Pierret, Mrs. E., 16
Pivar, David J., 149
pneumonia, 5, 25
police, 12, 17, 31, 118, 132, 144–146, 148–155, 188nn14,15, 189n24
police powers, 64, 67, 74–75, 124, 142
policewomen, 169n50
postnatal care, 104, 106, 111, 113, 122–126, 185–186n63
Pottenger, Francis Marion, 91, 94, 98–99, 101
poverty, 4, 157; and housing reform, 45, 50–51, 60, 62, 71; and midwifery/maternity programs, 111–113, 121, 124, 130; and milk reform, 88, 100; and public health nursing, 11, 14, 17, 24, 34–35, 42; and venereal disease programs, 139. *See also* immigrants; working classes
Powell, Lyman, 52
Powers, Luther Milton, 158; and housing reform, 54, 67, 73–74; and midwifery/maternity programs, 109, 117, 120, 126; and milk reform, 79, 82–84, 88–89, 91, 94, 98; and public health nursing, 10, 36–37, 41; and venereal disease programs, 136–137, 147, 149–150
pregnant women, 25, 104–109, *105,* 111–115, 119, 121–125, 130, 140. *See also* childbirth
premature birth, 109, 113
prenatal care, 104–106, 111, 113, 122–125, 185–186n63
Preston School of Industry, 148–149
prevention, 24, 145, 157
Price, Francis M., 34
price control, 82–84, 177n23
privacy, 72, 76, 133, 135
private funding, 12–15, 21, 38, 59, 68, 71
professionalism, 23–24, *23,* 27, 42, 110, 169n50

prostitution, 24, 49, 132–138, 143–145, 148–149, 151–154, 189nn22–25, 191–192n78

public health nursing, 7–9, 10–43, 159, 166n1; and Bethlehem Institute, 34–35; and Bureau of Municipal Nursing, 38, 41–43, 170n106; and College of Medicine, 33–35, 112; funding for, 10–15, 17–18, 20, 22, 25, 30, 40, 111, 114, 122, 156–157, 166n7; and gender factors, 26–27, 40–42, 170n106; and housing reform, 55–57, 59, 66, 68–69, 113; and measles epidemic, 37–40, 158; and midwifery/maternity programs, 104–105, *105*, 111–112, 115, 117, 120–124, 127–128, 130–131, 186n81; and nursing reports, 25–26, 28–32, *29*, 33–34, 36, 112–113; and public schools, 35–37, 40, 42–43; rules for, 22–24, 30, 111–112, 115, 131; statistics for, 18–20, 27–28, 35–36, 168n36, 169n69; and uniforms, 21, 23, *23,* 169n50; and venereal disease programs, 190n43; and Weston as supervisor, 20–28, *23,* 30, 34–39, 42, 111–115, 117, 120–124, 131, 168n37, 169n46

public schools, 35–37, 40, 42–43

puerperal fever, 108, 112

Pure Milk Campaign Committee, 94, 97, 99, 101–102

quackery, 25, 139, 141

quarantine, 37, 133–134, 147–149, 151, 154, 192n80

Quierolo, Nicholas, 67

race factors, 3, 5, 9, 20, 145, 159, 165n26; and housing reform, 45, 50, 56, 61–62; and midwifery/maternity programs, 106–107, 121, 123, 131, 182n6, 185n59. *See also* ethnicity

Red-Light Abatement Act (1913), 136–137

referendum, initiative, and recall, 3, 62, 178n43; and milk reform, 77–80, 86–87, 94, 96, 102 (*see also* tuberculin ordinance)

refrigerated transport, 92–93, 100

rehabilitation, 137, 145–147, 159, 192n80

religious groups, 5, 34, 101, 126, 130, 166n27. *See also names of religious denominations*

Reverby, Susan, 27

Reynolds, James Bronson, 6–8, 46, 157

Riis, Jacob, 8, 44–46, 49–54, 60, 66, 69, 74, 76, 157, 172nn21,30

Ritzer, George, 12

Rogers, Alfred R., 139–140, 187n6, 190n43

Rogers, Arthur M., 134, 140–141, 187n6

"Rooming-House Ordinance, The" (May 13, 1912), 136, 151–152, 188n15

Roosevelt, Theodore, 118

Rosenau, Milton J., 87

Rowland, Ward B., 90

Ruskin Art Club, 54

Russian immigrants, 1, 3, 159; and housing reform, 56, 61–62, 67, 69; and midwifery/maternity programs, 113, 123–124, 127; and public health nursing, 19, 25–26, 28–31, 35, 37

saloons, 46, 49, 116

Salvarsan, 135, 139–140, 143, 155, 158, 189n31

Salvation Army Rescue and Maternity Home, 114

sanitation, 2, 158; and housing reform, 45, 47–49, 52, 56–58, 60–61, 64, 66–68, 75; and midwifery/maternity programs, 111, 126; and milk reform, 79–82, 84, 92, 99; and public health nursing, 19, 25–26. *See also* hygienic practices

Schenck, Paul Wadsworth, 151, 153, 192n86

school nurses, 35–37, 40, 42–43

science, 8, 157–158; and housing reform, 45, 48, 57; and midwifery/maternity programs, 108, 111–112, 182n2; and milk reform, 78, 81–82, 85–86, 88–91, 94, 97–99, 101, 103; and public health nursing, 18, 22, 26–27, 30, 34, 41, 166n29; and venereal disease programs, 132, 134–135, 150–151, 192n85

Scott, H. W., 153

Second Ward, 10, 17, 33, 46, 50, 56, 113, 168n31. *See also* Sonoratown

Sedgwick, Mary K., 13

segregation, 5, 20, 113, 128

Seventh Ward, 46, 50, 168n31

Severance, Caroline, 6
sewage/water facilities, 2, 45, 48–49, 51, 57, 60–61, 64–65, 76, 143
Shaw, Judge Lucien, 12
Sheppard-Towner Maternity and Infancy Act (1920), 87
Sherman, Mina E., 95
Siewiecke, Louis, 12
Sirch, Margaret F., 40, 42, 124, 170n103, 186n81
Sixth Ward, 62–63, 174n63
slums, 8, 44–46, 50–52, 58, 63, 66, 76. *See also* house courts; tenements
smallpox, 4, 19, 37, 61
Smith, Catherine E., 109, 117–120, 184n46
Smith, Mary, 151–152
Sobieski, Lydia Gertrude, 95, 101, 180n86
social hygiene movement, 7, 134–136, 145, 155, 157, 191n61
socialism, 14–15, 78, 96–97, 100, 167n23
Sonoratown, 10, 47–50, 57
Southern California Practitioner, 98, 101, 108–109, 112, 139–140
Spalding, William A., 21
special nurses, 39–40, 42, 111, 124. *See also* maternity nurses
Spiker, Mary, 115–116
Stanley, Georgia, 146
Stetson, Jean, 153–154
Stoddart, Bessie, 57–58, 63
Stoddart, Evelyn, 10, 16, 172n34
Stoll, Alice, 79
Stout, J. F., 80–81
Straus, Nathan, 85, 89, 94, 103, 182n129
suffrage, 3–4, 46, 77–78, 85–86, 95–96, 136
sympathy, 8, 27, 30, 41, 78, 85, 134, 157, 166n29
syphilis, 132–133, 135–142, 155, 158, 188–189nn20,23

Taylor, Graham, 53–56, 157
telephone, 101, 122–123
Temple, Ruth Janetta, 123
tenements, 8; and housing reform, 44, 46–50, 52–53, 58, 60, 62, 64, 66–68, 72–75; and midwifery/maternity programs, 113; and public health nursing, 13, 35

Toll, Charles H., 11
Tomes, Nancy, 45
transportation of milk, 80, 84, 92–93, 100
tubercle bacillus, 90–91, 102
Tubercular Association, 40
tuberculin ordinance, 77–79, 85, 89, 91–103, 180n83, 181nn115,119
tuberculin testing, 77–78, 85–86, 90–95, 97–102, 178n43, 179n69
tuberculosis, 5, 61–62, 113, 147; and milk reform, 77, 85, 90–91, 94, 97–100; and public health nursing, 19, 26–27, 35, 40, 42–43
typhoid fever, 5, 19, 26, 49, 90
Typographical Union, 62

United Church Women of Los Angeles, 130
United Milk Producers Association, 94–95, 97–101
urbanization, 2–5, 7–8, 70; and midwifery/maternity programs, 107, 121–123, 185n59; and milk reform, 78–79, 82, 84–85, 87; and public health nursing, 16, 38, 45–46, 53
U.S. Bureau of the Census. *See* censuses
U.S. Department of Agriculture, 83, 90
U.S. Public Health Service (USPHS), 142
U.S. Supreme Court, 92–93, 102

vagrancy, 132–134, 148
Vecchio, Diane C., 182n2
Veeder, Mary Adair, 59–60, 173n49
Veiller, Lawrence, 62
venereal disease programs, 7–9, 112, 132–155, 159; and compulsory reporting, 133–135, 137; funding for, 141–143, 145, 149, 190n46; and Genito-Urinary Clinic, 134, 138–141, 190nn42,43; and Los Feliz Hospital, 133–134, 140–141, 143–150, *144*, 154–155, 190–191nn56,59; and prostitution, 24, 49, 132–138, 143–145, 148–149, 151–154, 189nn22–25, 191–192n78; and Salvarsan, 135, 139–140, 143, 155, 189n31; statistics for, 137–138, 140, 142–143, 147, 152, 188–189nn20,26; and World War I, 132, 134, 138, 141–145, 147–148, 152, 154–155, 190n44

Vestal, Thomas, 81
veterinarians, 90, 102
vice, 3, 49, 134–136, 139, 144, 147, 149, 151, 155, 188nn14,15. *See also* prostitution
visiting nurses, 13, 33, 190n43. *See also* public health nursing
volunteerism, 2, 5, 68, 74–75, 122–123
Von Wagner, Johanna, 69–73, *70,* 175n95

Wald, Lillian D., 13, 22
Wasserman, Augustus Paul von, 135
Wasserman tests, 134–135, 139, 150, 192n83
Waters, Isabella, 36, 168n36
Wellesley College, 7, 10, 21–22, 169n48
Weston, Maude Foster, 1, 20–28, *23,* 30, 34–39, 42, 169n46; and midwifery/maternity programs, 111–115, 117, 120–124, 131. *See also* Foster, Maude B.
Weston, Nathan, 20, 28, 168n38
whites, 5, 27, 50, 63, 86, 106, 112, 114, 118, 145, 148, 174n63. *See also* middle-class standards
whooping cough, 5, 19, 62
Wilbur, Curtis D., 138
Willard, Charles Dwight, 54, 58
Wilson, Zenobia Palmyra, 82–83, 177n23
Winslow, Kenelm, 89
Wise, Bessie, 119
Woman's City Club, 155
Woman's Court, 155
Woman's Hospital, 114
women. *See* gender factors; *entries beginning with* female
Women's Alliance Maternity Cottage, 114
Women's City Club, 96
Women's Civic Federation (WCF), 53–54, 56, 58, 172n34
women's rights, 95, 103, 136, 143, 145, 149. *See also* suffrage
Women's Sanitary Maternity Home, 114
Woods, Gerald, 164n11, 188n14
Woods, Robert A., 51
working classes, 1–4, 9, 156; and housing reform, 44–46, 51, 60, 63, 68, 74, 171n5; and midwifery/maternity programs, 104–106, *105,* 113–117, 183n29; and milk reform, 78–79, 86–87, 95–96, 101, 103; and public health nursing, 10–11, 16, 19, 24, 28–33; and venereal disease programs, 138–139, 145, 147–148, 188n8. *See also* immigrants
Workman, Mary J., 35, 166n27
World War I, 132, 134, 138, 141–145, 147–148, 152, 154–155, 190n44
Wright, C. W., 12

Young Women's Christian Association (YWCA), 22, 51

Zuber, Herman, 15–17
zymotic diseases, 5, 18. *See also* contagious diseases

About the Author

Jennifer Lisa Koslow received her Ph.D. from the University of California, Los Angeles. She is currently an assistant professor of history and director of Florida State University's Historical Administration and Public History Program.

Available titles in the Critical Issues in Health and Medicine series:

Emily K. Abel, *Suffering in the Land of Sunshine: A Los Angeles Illness Narrative*

Emily K. Abel, *Tuberculosis and the Politics of Exclusion: A History of Public Health and Migration to Los Angeles*

Susan M. Chambré, *Fighting for Our Lives: New York's AIDS Community and the Politics of Disease*

James Colgrove, Gerald Markowitz, and David Rosner, eds., *The Contested Boundaries of American Public Health*

Cynthia A. Connolly, *Saving Sickly Children: The Tuberculosis Preventorium in American Life, 1909–1970*

Edward J. Eckenfels, *Doctors Serving People: Restoring Humanism to Medicine through Student Community Service*

Julie Fairman, *Making Room in the Clinic: Nurse Practitioners and the Evolution of Modern Health Care*

Jill A. Fisher, *Medical Research for Hire: The Political Economy of Pharmaceutical Clinical Trials*

Gerald N. Grob and Howard H. Goldman, *The Dilemma of Federal Mental Health Policy: Radical Reform or Incremental Change?*

Gerald N. Grob and Allan V. Horwitz, *Diagnosis, Therapy, and Evidence: Conundrums in Modern American Medicine*

Laura D. Hirshbein, *American Melancholy: Constructions of Depression in the Twentieth Century*

Timothy Hoff, *Practice under Pressure: Primary Care Physicians and Their Medicine in the Twenty-first Century*

Rebecca M. Kluchin, *Fit to Be Tied: Sterilization and Reproductive Rights in America, 1950–1980*

Jennifer Lisa Koslow, *Cultivating Health: Los Angeles Women and Public Health Reform*

Bonnie Lefkowitz, *Community Health Centers: A Movement and the People Who Made It Happen*

Ellen Leopold, *Under the Radar: Cancer and the Cold War*

Barbara L. Ley, *From Pink to Green: Disease Prevention and the Environmental Breast Cancer movement*

David Mechanic, *The Truth about Health Care: Why Reform Is Not Working in America*

Alyssa Picard, *Making the American Mouth: Dentists and Public Health in the Twentieth Century*

Karen Seccombe and Kim A. Hoffman, *Just Don't Get Sick: Access to Health Care in the Aftermath of Welfare Reform*

Leo B. Slater, *War and Disease: Biomedical Research on Malaria in the Twentieth Century*

Rosemary A. Stevens, Charles E. Rosenberg, and Lawton R. Burns, eds., *History and Health Policy in the United States: Putting the Past Back In*

Printed in the United States
219833BV00001B/1/P